W9-AXQ-667

PRAISE FOR
TERRY HOPE ROMERO

"For salad inspiration, I can think of few sources better than the new cookbook *Salad Samurai*. . . . Romero brings her fun-loving sensibility and unerring palate to the table. Her recipes, with their brilliant combinations, span the seasons."

—*Washington Post*

"We've all heard the dreaded 'but where do you get your protein?' question, and thanks to Terry Hope Romero, we've now got answers, as the vegan icon's latest cookbook features 100 plant-protein-packed recipes perfect for everyone from professional athletes to people on the go."

—*VegNews*

"Romero rounds up a big world of fusion and flavors for 100 cutting-edge salads. . . . *Salad Samurai* recipes are bold, but totally doable. Romero gives you the recipes as well as their individual components from spirited dressings to crunchy, cool toppings, so you can mix, match and tap into your own inner salad samurai."

—*Huffington Post*

"With creative and satisfying recipes, including ones that are gluten free and nut free, Romero's latest is sure to be in demand for eaters of all types, especially those who avoid eating animal products."

—*Library Journal*

"If you're ready to take your salads to the next level, Terry Hope Romero offers all kinds of ideas in *Salad Samurai*. . . . Along with a plethora of amazing and tempting recipes, Romero has also included a generous helping of the lively wit that her readers adore. Anyone familiar with her past cookbooks won't be surprised to learn that every recipe in *Salad Samurai* is vegan, but don't let that scare you away; there's a recipe in this book for everyone."

—*San Francisco Book Review*

"Full of complex, belly-filling, sometimes even show-stopping meals that happen to be salads. And vegan . . . *Salad Samurai* is something of a wonder."

—SeriousEats.com

"Includes 100 recipes . . . that prove that salads are a lot more than what you have to eat before the real meal comes."

—*LA Weekly*

"Its accessible main course salad recipes are anything but boring, with unexpected flavor combinations that make me wonder—hey, why didn't I think of that?"

—Epicurious.com

"Creative salad offerings. . . . Color photos and helpful tips can be found throughout this book."

—*Vegetarian Journal*

"*Salad Samurai* will prove to be an invaluable, 'kitchen cook friendly' addition to all personal, family, and community library cookbook collections. . . . Beautifully illustrated throughout. . . . Especially recommended for parents of children reluctant to eat a salad and for anyone trying to establish healthy eating habits."

—Midwest Book Review

"If you hunger for satisfying, plant-based meals instead of demure side-dish salads, this book is for you!"

—Taste for Life

"*Protein Ninja* deliciously explains how to sneak more protein into vegan recipes."

—*Vegetarian Times*

SHOW UP FOR SALAD

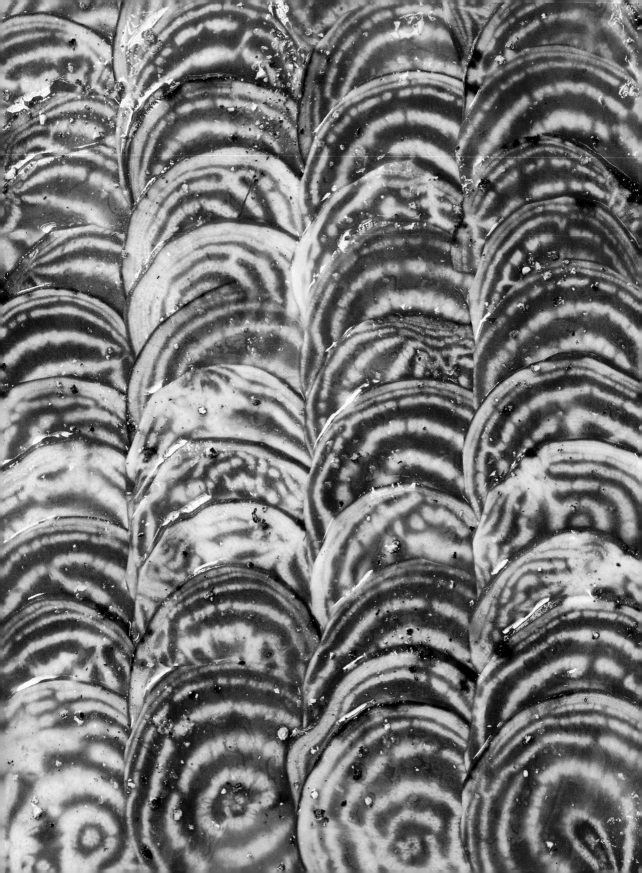

TERRY HOPE ROMERO

100 More Recipes FOR SALADS, DRESSINGS & ALL THE FIXINS...

SHOW UP FOR SALAD

...YOU DON'T HAVE TO BE VEGAN to Love!

Da Capo
LIFE LONG

The information in this book is true and complete to the best of our knowledge. This book is intended only as an informative guide for those wishing to know more about health issues. In no way is this book intended to replace, countermand, or conflict with the advice given to you by your own physician. The ultimate decision concerning care should be made between you and your doctor. We strongly recommend you follow his or her advice. Information in this book is general and is offered with no guarantees on the part of the authors or Da Capo Press. The authors and publisher disclaim all liability in connection with the use of this book. The names and identifying details of people associated with events described in this book have been changed. Any similarity to actual persons is coincidental.

Many of the designations used by manufacturers and sellers to distinguish their products are claimed as trademarks. Where those designations appear in this book and Da Capo Press was aware of a trademark claim, the designations have been printed in initial capital letters.

Copyright © 2019 by Terry Hope Romero

Cover design by Shubhani Sarkar, sarkardesignstudio.com
Cover photograph by Vanessa K. Rees
Cover copyright © 2019 Hachette Book Group, Inc.

Hachette Book Group supports the right to free expression and the value of copyright. The purpose of copyright is to encourage writers and artists to produce the creative works that enrich our culture.

The scanning, uploading, and distribution of this book without permission is a theft of the author's intellectual property. If you would like permission to use material from the book (other than for review purposes), please contact permissions@hbgusa.com. Thank you for your support of the author's rights.

Da Capo Press
Hachette Book Group
1290 Avenue of the Americas, New York, NY 10104
www.dacapopress.com
@DaCapoPress

Printed in the United States of America

First Edition: June 2019

Published by Da Capo Press, an imprint of Perseus Books, LLC, a subsidiary of Hachette Book Group, Inc.

The Hachette Speakers Bureau provides a wide range of authors for speaking events. To find out more, go to www.hachettespeakersbureau.com or call (866) 376-6591.

The publisher is not responsible for websites (or their content) that are not owned by the publisher.

Photos by Vanessa K. Rees
Print book interior design by Shubhani Sarkar, sarkardesignstudio.com

Library of Congress Cataloging-in-Publication Data
Names: Romero, Terry Hope, author.
Title: Show up for salad: 100 more recipes for salads, dressings, and all the fixins you don't have to be vegan to love / Terry Hope Romero.
Description: First edition. | New York, NY: Da Capo Press, 2019. | Includes index.
Identifiers: LCCN 2018047188| ISBN 9780738218519 (pbk.) | ISBN 9780738218526 (ebook)
Subjects: LCSH: Salads. | Vegan cooking.
Classification: LCC TX807 .R65 2019 | DDC 641.83—dc23
LC record available at https://lccn.loc.gov/2018047188

ISBNs: 978-0-73821-851-9 (paperback), 978-0-73821-852-6 (ebook)

LSC-C

10 9 8 7 6 5 4 3 2 1

To everyone making vegan choices every day
(from what they eat, to what they wear,
to how they spend their time and resources)
to save our health, our precious environment,
and the lives of farm animals

CONTENTS

INTRODUCTION: CHOOSE YOUR OWN SALAD ADVENTURE *1*

SLAY THAT SALAD *3*

CHOOSING & STORING GREENS & VEGGIES *5*

FIVE KITCHEN TOOLS FOR SALAD SEEKERS *7*

THE SALAD PANTRY: EVERYTHING BUT THE VEGGIES *11*

DIY MICROGREENS: A PARTIAL GUIDE *14*

SALADS FOR NERDS: HOW TO MAKE SALAD WITH A SCALE *19*

STASH THAT SALAD *20*

TO THE GLUTEN-FREE, NUT-FREE, SOY-FREE SALAD ENTHUSIAST *21*

THE RECIPES

DRESSINGS AND TOPPINGS
smartly dressed salads

DRESSINGS

THE ZEN OF HEMP DRESSING

Hemp Seed Caesar Dressing 31

Hemp Seed Tarragon Dijon Dressing 32

Creamy Italian Hemp Dressing 33

Horseradish Hemp Dressing 34

THE WAY OF SUNFLOWER SEED DRESSINGS

Sunflower Ranch Dressing 37

Sun and Sea Sunflower Caesar Dressing 39

Sriracha Cilantro Ranch Dressing 40

TAHINI-BASED CREAMY DRESSINGS

Tahini Mayo 43

Turmeric Tahini Miso Sauce 44

Tahini French Dressing 45

Oil-Free Cashew Lemon Pepper Dressing 46

Cucumber Dill Dressing 48

Pepita Greenest Goddess Dressing 51

Red Pepper and Almond Romesco Dressing 52

Sultry Peanut Coconut Dressing 54

Deep Dark Sesame Dressing 55

Wasabi Miso Lime Dressing 56

Ginger Garlic Fire Dressing 57

Carrot Ginger Dressing 58

Roasted Pico de Gallo Dressing 59

Sun-Dried Tomato Dressing 60

Hollyhock Dressing 61

New Catalina Dressing 62

Salted Lemons 64

1-MINUTE VINAIGRETTES FOR EVERY DAY

Keep It Simple Vinaigrette 67

Bright and Tangy Lemon
Maple Vinaigrette 68

Oregano Garlic Lemon Vinaigrette 69

Maple Mustard Shallot Vinaigrette 70

Balsamic Dijon Vinaigrette 71

The Best Orange Balsamic Vinaigrette 72

SAVORY PLANT-BASED PROTEIN TOPPINGS

MIGHTY AND FLAVORFUL
TOFU, TEMPEH, AND SEITAN

Marinated Baked Tofu 75

Fried or Grilled Tofu 76

Marinated or Baked Tempeh 77

Marinated Pan-Fried Seitan 78

Marinated Roasted Yuba 79

Marinated Pan-Fried Aburaage 80

Steamed Seitan Cutlets 81

THE MARINADES

Hot Sauce Buffalo 84

Savory Sesame Tamari 85

Korean BBQ 86

Peruvian Chile Lime 87

Lemon Dijon 89

Sriracha Orange 90

Sweet Lime Curry 91

Tahini Miso 92

Golden Coriander Bird 93

Maple Almost Like Bacon 94

Oven-Fried Breakfast Tofu Bites 95

Whole-Loaf Blackened Tempeh Pastrami 97

Roasted Lemon Pepper Chickpeas 100

Salt-and-Pepper Fried White Beans 102

SALAD RICE, DRESSED LENTILS,
OR OTHER GRAINS OR BEANS

Dressed Lentils 104

Salad Rice 105

Homemade Beans 106

Quinoa for Salad 108

NUTTY, CHEESY, CRUNCHY TOPPINGS

Toasted Sun and Pepita Parm 110

7-Spice Peanuts 111

Crumbly, Salty Almond Cheese 113

Crispy, Cheesy Almond Crunch 117

Nut-Free, Soy-Free
Cheesy Sunflower Crunch 118

BACON CRUNCH NUTS AND SEEDS

Bacon Crunch Hazelnuts 121

Bacon Crunch Pecans 121

Sweet and Salty Pecans 121

Caesar Walnuts 123

CRISPY, CHEWY VEGGIE TOPPINGS

Maple Mushroom Bacon 125

Root Bacon 127

Pastrami Carrots 130

Beet Prosciutto 131

Pan-Roasted Chile Corn 134

Crispy Lime-and-Salt Shallots 135

Red Onion Quick Pickle 136

CROUTONS AND TOASTY BITES

Savory Coconut Chips, 3 Ways 138

    Chipotle Bacon 138

    Coconut Turmeric Lime 138

    Salt, Pepper, and Vinegar 138

Seedy Garlic Bread Croutons 139

    Basil Pesto Croutons 140

    Simple Croutons 140

    Naked Toasts 140

No-Oil Chia Crunch Croutons 141

Cheesy, Crispy Croutons 142

Herbed Cornbread Crunch 145

Vegan Cornbread Loaf 146

Sweet, Salty, Nutty Gomasio 148

THE SALADS

GREEN, CRISPY, CRUNCHY, CHEWY

The Bright and Spicy Spring
Asparagus Salad 151

The Juicy Grilled Summer Days
Peach Salad 155

The Big Crunchy Autumn Vibes Salad 159

The Bold and Bountiful Winter Salad 160

Forever Kale Caesar
with Cheesy, Crispy Croutons 163

    Classic Romaine Caesar 164

    Restaurant-Style Entrée Caesar 164

Sriracha Ranch Salad Party 165

    Salad Pizza 166

Sriracha Tofu Lettuce Wraps
with Peanut Dressing 169

Chickpea Pickle Collard Wraps 170

Orange Collard Greens, Corn,
and Black-Eyed Peas 173

Buffalo Tofu, Butternut Squash,
and Kale Bowl 176

Blackened Tempeh Reuben Salad 179

ROASTED, GRILLED, AND HEARTY SALADS

Thai Basil Spaghetti Squash
with Curry Tofu 181

General Tso's Tofu and Broccoli Salad 185

Roasted Cabbage Steak
with Peanut Sauce and Fried Shallots 186

Roasted Niçoise Salad 188

Protein-Packed Salad for Breakfast 191

All-Day Breakfast Nacho Salad Bowl 192

Kabocha and Black Rice Salad 195

    Green Curry Paste 196

White Sweet Potato Salad with
Spinach Zhug Dressing 198

Roasted Ratatouille Salad
with Romesco Dressing   201

Lazy Seitan Gyro Spinach Salad   204

Crunchy Eggplant Parm Salad   207

PASTA AND GRAINS WITH GREENS

Peanut Avocado Brown Rice
Crunch Bowl   211

Spicy Cucumber and Curry Tofu Salad with
Sticky Rice   212

   Steamed Sticky Rice   215

Peking-Roasted Tofu Noodle Salad   217

Korean Shiitake Bacon Salad Rice Bowl   219

   Gochujang Dressing   221

Mustard Greens Tabbouleh
with Almonds and Roasted Chickpeas   222

Peruvian Potato and Red Quinoa Salad   225

Charred Broccoli, Potato,
and Root Bacon Salad   229

Roasted Tomato Chickpea Pasta Salad   231

Pizza Panzanella with Beet Prosciutto   235

Zucchini and Chickpea Fattoush Salad   237

Greek Golden Fava Salad Pita   241

Avocado and Black Bean Salad
on Cornbread Toast   243

SOUP MEETS SALAD

Potato Leek Soup with
Broccoli Gremolata   247

Buffalo Tomato Soup
with Kale Caesar Salad   250

Green Again Soup with Tahini Miso Slaw   253

Creamy Cauliflower Soup
with Apple Walnut Salad   254

Ethiopian Red Lentils with Butternut
and Avocado Collard Salad   257

Baby Carrot Ginger Soup
with Sesame Slaw   260

Cranberry Bean and Pasta Stew
with Fennel Slaw   262

Thai Peanut Curry
with Quick Cucumber Pickles   265

Veggie Noodle Pho with
Micro Bahn Mi Salad   267

Red Lentil Khichdi with Two Chutneys   269

White Bean and Seitan Green Posole
with Avocado Radish Salad   273

METRIC CONVERSION CHART   275

ACKNOWLEDGMENTS   277

INDEX   279

ABOUT THE AUTHOR   291

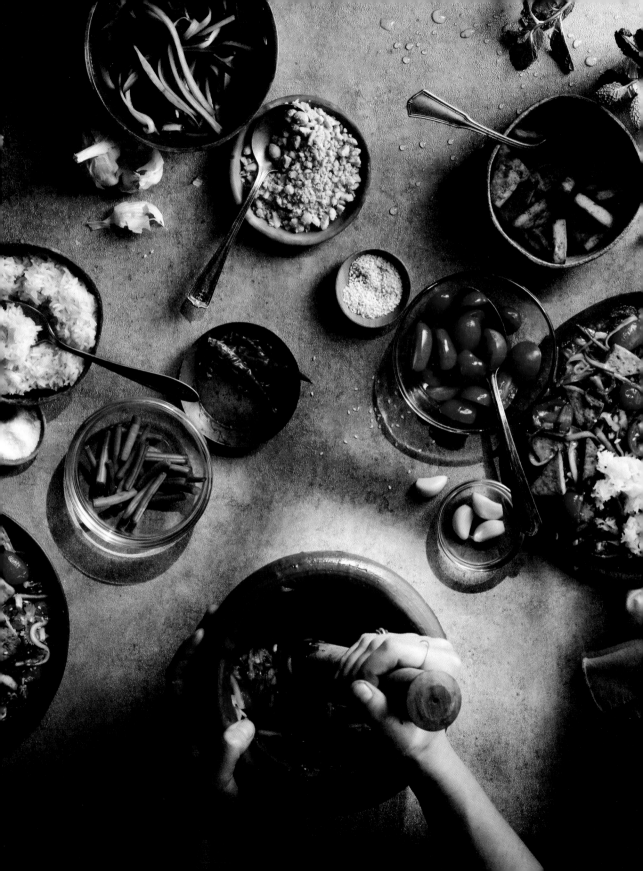

INTRODUCTION
Choose Your Own Salad Adventure

The unmistakably hearty, filling, and entirely vegan salad (and soup) recipes in this book are designed to be enjoyed à la carte. Go ahead and cherry-pick to your heart's content. A dressing on Tuesday night, a tasty tofu to garnish veggies after work, a complete dressed salad for a chill Saturday night dinner, or just some "cheesy" croutons to drop on your own fast salad or even a soup. My hope is that you'll create a highly customized salad bar that excites *your* palate. It's a DIY salad bar that awaits when you open the refrigerator wondering, *What's to eat?* so you can show up for salad every damn day.

First step? Stock the fridge with a few Dressings and Toppings (page 25). At the store, grab the best-looking greens and vegetables, open the fridge, pull out a homemade dressing, and whip up a zesty flavored tofu in the oven while you wash, spin, and chop the produce. Once the tofu (or whatever topping) is ready, it's just a matter of dressing it all, piling into big bowls, and maybe garnishing with uniquely tasty croutons or crunchy roasted nuts made by you. It's that easy.

Ah, but lest you still think, *Eh, salad is not a meal,* my friend, listen up. Flavorful and filling salad toppings are my specialty. I'm not gonna let you go hungry. Even after a decade of vegan cookbook writing, I still believe that tofu, tempeh, and seitan are the most accessible and interesting ways to include filling and wholesome protein into meatless meals. Pair them with legumes (a.k.a. beans and lentils, a.k.a. the other crucial vegan protein), and you are well on your way to insanely hearty salads. But don't think that's all that can top your salad; there's a whole world of entirely plant-based options (beet prosciutto, parsnip, or carrot bacon . . .).

And what's salad without dressing? Dressings enhance, garnish, and enliven. They transform naked, raw, or simple roasted produce into meals. For most of us, a salad is defined entirely by what it's poured with or tossed with. There are clean and sharp vinaigrettes, and rich and silky seed- and nut-based dressings, and a few in-between concoctions that get their body and substance from helpful ingredients like sun-dried tomatoes or mustards. Once you discover how great and easy homemade dressings are, you'll find it hard to savor a store-bought dressing ever again.

I know there are days where you don't want to make it up. You just want a recipe that tells you what to eat. Be still; I've still got you covered there too. The "complete" recipes (salad and soup, garnished with small salads) are ones that show up for you—you can make 'em as is; they also serve as inspiration to create your combinations. They are the sum of their parts; choose a dressing, make a topping or two, then toss them together with the main attractions: the greens, the vegetables and fruits, or grains, beans, pastas, potatoes. They can be followed to the letter (or used as maps for off-road adventures, inspirations for your own creations). We will all show up for salad in our own way.

SLAY THAT SALAD

The main salad recipes in this book refer to other recipes (dressings and toppings) to pull it all together. To make the most out of your kitchen time, I suggest preparing those smaller recipes in the following order:

FIRST

Check the pantry and fridge to see what you already have in stock. Maybe you already invested in great olive oil or have a massive box of kosher salt. Soak any nuts to be used for dressings. Simply cover with about 2 inches of warm water in a covered glass container and set on the kitchen counter for 30 minutes or up to 3 hours until the nuts are soft and plump. Different nuts require different soaking, with raw cashews needing less than an hour and almonds up to 3 or more. Or if you'd rather sleep than ponder soaking nuts, let them soak covered and overnight in the fridge.

MAKE THE DRESSING

After presoaked seeds or nuts, most dressings take just minutes to prepare and can rest in the fridge while you do the rest.

MAKE THE TOPPINGS

Roast or cook the toppings. Bread- and vegetable-based toppings recipes in this book such as croutons make a lot, suitable for many salads, so this step will likely set you up with enough for a few recipes.

WASH, SPIN, CHOP

Wash and spin dry the greens, then seal them in an airtight container and keep chilled. If your greens are very fresh (like plucked from the ground that morning kind of fresh), try this method to keep them lively for a week or more: snugly wrap freshly washed yet dripping wet greens in a clean kitchen towel, then loosely wrap in produce bags and store in the fridge. The towel will dampen, wrapping crisp, fresh greens and protecting them from the drying environment of the fridge.

Dice or slice chunky, hard fresh veggies (broccoli, cauliflower, squash, peppers, carrots, green beans) and remove the seeds (if necessary), and store them in the fridge until it's time to make the salad.

Tomatoes, potatoes, and eggplants are best sliced just prior to preparing (roasting, serving, etc.), as nightshades brown and get weepy as soon as you slice 'em.

ASSEMBLE AND SERVE

It's salad showtime! Assemble salad on a platter or a pan for eaters to shovel onto their own plates, or just make one serving at a time for individual servings. Start by layering fluffy greens first, then heap on vegetables, grains, and croutons. Drizzle with a little dressing and toss to coat elements with dressing goodness. Layer the proteins on top and scatter on garnishes like chopped herbs or crunchy nuts and seeds. Drizzle with a little more dressing, and pass around any remaining dressing for people to enjoy as they will. Beautiful salads *do* taste as good as they look.

MISE EN SALAD (OR MISE EN PLACE FOR SALADS)

Mise en place simply put means "everything in its place." In practice, every ingredient is prepared and placed in discrete little bowls. If you're new to the practice, making yet another cluster of dirty dishes may feel daunting, yet when juggling a list of ingredients, mise en place (hopefully) will prevent any forgotten steps when following a new recipe.

The method is straightforward: clean, chop, measure, and set aside each ingredient *before* combining together. It's helpful to put each ingredient into its own cup and line up in the order of adding to the mixing bowl. Clearly seeing each ingredient creates a no-goof road map for the final recipe. This can take many forms; I'll usually line up my little parade of pinch bowls and cups around the edge of the cutting board or assemble wedges of chopped vegetables on a dinner plate.

When I'm lacking a dozen little bowls, I'll group together the small stuff, like all the ground spices in the same cup or tablespoons of vinegars or juices together in a bowl. Maybe that would flunk me out of cooking school, but it's a version of mise en place that works in a pinch.

CHOOSING & STORING GREENS & VEGGIES

I'll bet you a hundred baby carrots you can spy a fresh-looking vegetable when you see it: firm, bright color, and relatively heavy. The longer vegetables and fruit sit around, the more water they lose, and they start to look shriveled and feel lighter. Greens of all kinds follow the same patterns: look for firm, sturdy leaves and avoid heavily wilted leaves with many yellow or brown patches.

Buying prewashed salad greens in bags or boxes (they are very convenient and, yes, sometimes the best-looking option in the store)? Look at the bottom of the box or bag, through any writing on the package, and skip packages with limp or crushed leaves clumped at the bottom. Chances are these greens are past their prime. If in doubt about the age of washed, packaged greens at home, give them the smell test! Fresh (or fresh enough) greens should smell clean and sweet; older, on-their-way-out greens will have that certain rotten aroma. Yuck! Time to order a pizza! Or instead of a green salad, make a filling grain- or roasted vegetable–based salad instead.

SOAKING GREENS

It happens to everyone. You buy a beautiful bunch of kale on Sunday. In a hurry, it goes into the veggie bin in the fridge. By Thursday, life finally slows down enough to make that kale Caesar salad, and those beautiful greens—while still green—are just tired, flabby, and limp.

A deep soak in very cold water will perk up those sad greens! Kale, collards, even tender leaves such as spinach or arugula will firm up when submerged in a big bowl of very cold water for about twenty minutes. Add a few ice cubes if the water isn't quite cold enough. Drain and spin dry just before making the salad.

WASHING AND DRYING GREENS

Wash every and all greens with plenty of cold water. Fluffy greens and many fresh herbs (such as basil) often come with plenty of sand, great on beaches but unpleasant when biting into a salad. I even wash "triple washed" packaged greens when they look less than stand-up fresh or if there's any question they may be starting to get a little soft.

By far the easiest way to wash greens at home is with a large salad spinner; any variety should have a colander-like inside that can be used to swish greens around and drain fast. For easy, fast cleaning, I prefer to chop greens, then wash. No salad spinner? Find a huge mixing bowl and cover greens with cold water, swish for a few minutes, then drain. Transfer to a colander to shake away large blobs of water. See, it's already double the work without a spinner.

Next, dry the greens. Why bother drying washed greens at all? Dressings and vinaigrettes just slide off wet greens, and all that water just dilutes the flavor of the salad. A salad spinner does it in a flash. No spinner still? Gently spread the greens over a large clean kitchen towel. Now roll up the towel, just like rolling up a jelly roll. Gently squeeze the towel roll and repeat again if the greens are still very wet. (But really, get yourself a salad spinner. Totally worth it.)

FIVE KITCHEN TOOLS
FOR SALAD SEEKERS

Good tools are essential for making better salads. No matter if you fancy yourself an artist crafting an elegant repast or a handy person bolting dinner together— these tools are essentials in the kitchen rather than simply nice to have. Yes, you can make some kind of salad without them, but your salad-making game will be so much more productive, fun, and rewarding with a Japanese mandoline or a knife sharp enough to slice a tomato. Worried about breaking the bank for salad? Most of the tools below will last you—and you can get most of them for a reasonable price. And you may already have some version of these essentials lurking in your kitchen!

(ACTUALLY SHARP) KITCHEN KNIVES

Chef's Knife (8- or 10-inch blade)

If you've been cutting vegetables up to this point with an ancient steak knife, get ready to have your mind blown. Chef's knives, when properly maintained, will transform your slow and tedious country-roads chopping into an express HOV superhighway breaking-the-speed-limit chopping. While you're at it, get yourself a knife steel (the thing that looks like a Teenage Mutant Ninja Turtle weapon); this does not sharpen the blade but keeps the knife edge straighter for cleaner slicing.

A great knife should not cost more than a new sofa. Quality knives can run between thirty and fifty dollars, have a blade than runs the entire length of the handle, and feel heavy and balanced in your dominant hand. Chef's knives are designed to rock on the cutting board. The blade should stay in constant contact with the surface. Scour your local T.J. Maxx or Marshalls for discounted knives, or get a knife from my friends at Misen (misen.co), who have made it their mission to create excellent business-class knives (and cookware!) at economy-seating prices.

After you get that knife, learn how to use it. For the most control of you knife, place your thumb on the base of the blade and not just the top of the handle. YouTube is full of great knife skills videos, or see the Misen site (yet again) for some nice displays of chef's knives in action.

Santoku Knife

Santoku are classic Japanese kitchen knives, as effective and ranging wildly in price as chef's knives. Santoku knives have a shorter, wider blade with a rather flat edge, unlike the curved edge of a western knife. If you would rather *chop chop chop chop* things up and down, instead of scissor rocking back and forth on the cutting board, then consider a santoku knife. Many santoku knife blades have the handy feature of a granton edge (shallow divots near the blade), which help prevent hard, starchy vegetables (potatoes, carrots) from gluing themselves to the blade while slicing. There are beautiful knives with blades rippled like samurai swords that cost hundreds, but you can attack salad recipes effectively with a budget santoku under twenty dollars.

Sharp Knives Spare the Tomato

A heavy knife with a really sharp edge practically cuts vegetables for you. It's a pity when a good knife is too dull to effortlessly slice a tomato. Hear me out: You are far more likely to cut yourself working with a dull blade than a sharp blade (dull blades can slide from vegetables onto fingers faster than you can blink). Respect your wrists, your knuckles, and hard-earned produce and learn how to keep your kitchen knives sharp. I use a simple sharpening tool (less than ten dollars on Amazon.com) for knife-edge upkeep about once every few weeks. A few times a year, I take my hardworking knives to a professional knife sharpener for a hard-core sharpening. Your salads will look, and even taste, all the better for it!

Y-SHAPED PEELERS (STRAIGHT BLADE, SERRATED, JULIENNE PEELER)

In the eternal struggle to determine which vegetable peeler is best, the Y-shaped peeler wins every time. Great for tired hands, achy hands, big hands and small, the Y-shaped peeler is much more pleasant to use than the standard stick peeler.

The Kuhn Rikon Swiss peeler is worth the hype and the same peelers have lived in my kitchen for years and still blast vegetables to shreds. Beyond the standard blade, a serrated blade is ideal for skinning hard winter squash or bumpy-skinned roots like celeriac. For salads, a julienne blade peeler (with large grooves) creates long, elegant threads of carrot, daikon, cucumber, and the like that are more attractive on salads than the stubby, flat shreds that fall out of a box grater.

SALAD SPINNER

I've been asked what's the most-used gadget in my kitchen, and beyond a knife, it may be a salad spinner. Beside drying soft, tender greens perfectly, it's the ideal thing to wash nearly every vegetable or fruit from kale to blueberries. There are cute little spinners for cleaning 3 lettuce leaves at a time; skip these in favor of the biggest spinner you can fit on your shelf; a 3-quart spinner is the standard for cleaning greens for 3 to 4 servings.

A HUGE STAINLESS STEEL
MIXING BOWL (OR A FEW)

I've cooked in the kitchens of friends and strangers the world over and often just down the street from my home, and the one thing overall that most people lack (after a suitable kitchen knife) are big mixing bowls! A big bowl, the kind you could cradle a small watermelon starting at about 14 inches wide, is highly effective for making a big salad. They are annoyingly hard to find! I have a set of stainless steel bowls from IKEA's BLANDA line that after years of cooking look as good as the day I got them, even after making many, many, many salads (and a lifetime of bread and pizza dough for parties too). If you see big stainless steel bowls (or something similar), get them and hold on to them like your salad-making life depends on it.

LONG-HANDLED TONGS

Another item I can't find salad happiness without and, like everything else in this list, can be purchased for next to nothing and made out of materials build to last. Pick up a pair or two of stainless steel tongs and get ready to combine salad like a pro!

TOOLS OF HONORABLE MENTION

Japanese Mandoline

Not your mother's or your brother's French cooking school mandoline! The Japanese mandoline was a revelation to me. I knew well the proper French mandoline—a massive, heavy tool from my ancient cooking school days that cost upward of $300. Hated it. Years later, with a Japanese mandoline in my life, this incredibly useful kitchen tool has changed my salad life unlike any other gadget.

This slim, lightweight, easy-to-store, simple-to-clean device runs about forty dollars. Translucent slivers of daikon or paper-thin slices of zucchini, beets, radishes, and piles of needle-thin cucumber matchsticks slide out of this thing in an instant. The blades are still sword-edge sharp and deserve the same respect as a French mandoline, but cleaning and storing a Japanese mandoline will feel like second nature. Benriner is the brand of choice; steer clear of cheap and flimsy knockoffs. My little "green knob" older-model Benriner mandoline has shredded me through this salad book along with mountains of cucumber and papaya salad meals.

Mason Jars

If you've ever seen food on Instagram, you know what a mason jar is, but it is worth the mention that quart widemouthed jars are my go-to storage setup. German mason jars are beautiful and interesting, but I find the combination of a rubber gasket, metal clips, and easy-to-chip glass lid too fussy and fragile to bother with.

High-Powered Blenders and Immersion Blenders

Smooth, creamy dressings need a quality blender to get the job done. I love my Blendtec blender with the extremely effective Twister Jar top: The "arms" of the jar lid scrape down the sides of the jar with minimal effort from you. For a more budget-friendly option, consider the Ninja blender. An immersion blender (stick blender) is my sidearm of choice for puréeing soups and making the occasional dressing too. I don't use food processors often, with the exception of a mini food processor for attacking small batches of chunky dressings or sauces.

THE SALAD PANTRY
Everything but the Veggies

The following pantry items appear throughout recipes in this book. They're shelf stable and typically sold in generous portions to stretch into many recipes, so grab them on your next shopping trip and don't be surprised when you find uses for them in many recipes.

Vinegars: Essential for dressing salads. A bottle of **apple cider, red wine, sherry,** and **white wine vinegars** will last through many salads.

Oils: **Extra-virgin olive oil** and **grape-seed oil** are my preferred oils for vinaigrettes. On occasion, I may use deep green **avocado oil** or mellow **walnut oil** in place of grape-seed oil (they are expensive oils but an affordable luxury). **Virgin coconut oil** and **refined coconut oil** (coconut oil refined just enough to remove the coconut aroma) show up in a few tofu recipes and soups in this book.

Dried herbs: The standard jars of dried **basil, dill, garlic powder, onion flakes, oregano,** and **thyme** are used in many of these recipes.

Spices: **Anaheim chili powder, black pepper (ground and whole kernel), cayenne pepper, chipotle chili powder, cumin, curry power, paprika (hot, sweet, and smoked), mustard powder,** and **turmeric** are essential. A few spice blends are also used in many recipes, including **Chinese 5-spice powder, Indian garam masala,** and **Ethiopian berbere.** If you can't find these blends, I've included my version of these spice blends too!

Nuts and seeds: I use plenty of **unroasted cashews, sesame seeds (roasted, unhulled), sunflower, sliced almonds, walnuts, pepitas (hulled pumpkin seeds), shelled hemp seeds,** and **chia seeds,** which are essential for creamy dressings and crunchy toppings, in these recipes.

Canned: Pantry staples of beans and tomatoes boost the flavor and nutritional content of many salads! Pick up a few cans of **black beans, chickpeas, black-eyed peas, tomato paste,** and **diced tomatoes (plain and fire roasted).**

Dried legumes: While they require a little more planning, nothing beats the flavor of homemade beans. A bag of **cranberry beans, green lentils, black lentils, French lentils, red lentils,** and **sprouted mung beans** go into many recipes in this book.

Condiments: Most are refrigerated, and a little goes a long way. These recipes make good use of **Dijon mustard, hoisin sauce, tamari, wasabi prepared paste or powder, white or yellow miso,** and **sriracha hot sauce.**

Salt: I am picky about salt! **Diamond (brand) kosher salt** is a flaky, crunchy, lightly textured salt I use for these recipes (see A Word from the Salt Box, page 13).

ETHNIC MARKETS

These pantry items can be found in some larger grocery chains and natural food stores but are sometimes cheaper in ethnic markets.

Black sesame seeds: Black sesame seeds have a firm bite and a slightly smoky flavor, and they look great sprinkled on any Asian salad.

Gojuchang (Korean red pepper paste) and Korean red pepper powder: There's simply no substitute for the mellow heat of Korean red pepper products. Gojuchang is thick, sweetened paste made from fermented chiles; if you love sriracha, you'll be a fan of gojuchang! Korean red pepper powder are fine flakes with mild fruity heat. *Do not* substitute with red pepper flakes.

Thai bird chiles (Asian, Thai): When it comes to really hot Asian chiles, slim red Thai bird wins every time. Full of flavor along with spark, a small bag will last through many salads. One or two chiles is usually enough for an entire dish.

Soba noodles: This ever-popular buckwheat noodle makes for fantastic summery salads. Udon noodles (wheat noodles) also are regularly on my shopping list.

Sumac powder (Middle Eastern): This maroon powder with a unique sweet-and-sour flavor is made from ground sumac berries. A dusting over salads just before serving adds a final punch of flavor.

Vinegar, rice: A mild, versatile white vinegar that's another staple in my pantry of vinegars. Great for adding tang to Asian marinades and dressings.

NATURAL FOODS

As the line between natural and mainstream grocery stores continues to blur, you'll likely find these items in some mainstream, well-stocked markets.

Nutritional yeast: The essential vegan food that adds umami, cheesy flavor to so many recipes. If possible, buy it in bulk or by the bagful; this is an ingredient and not just a sprinkle-on condiment. For an added boost of B12, look for brands labeled *vegetarian support formula.*

Seaweeds (also common in Asian markets): There's a little bit of seaweed in this book, mostly sushi-grade sheets of **nori.** If you're looking to add a little ocean flavor to a dressing, look for powdered **arame** or **wakame** seaweed.

Tamari: Japanese-style soy sauce that adds salty richness to so many vegan recipes. Grab a bottle of organic or low-sodium or gluten-free tamari, if desired.

Tofu: For the array of tofu recipes you'll soon dig into, use only firm or extra-firm water-packed (Chinese style). *Note: I don't use silken shelf-stable boxed tofu in this book.*

Tempeh: The firm and nutty fermented soybean cake that's great grilled, baked, or pan-fried. If you have access to fresh, locally made tempeh, then by all means try it with these recipes.

Seitan: The "meat from wheat" is a gluten lover's best friend when it comes to hearty, chewy meat substitutes. You can make your own simple steamed version at home (page 81) or use a ready-to-eat, plain, or flavored seitan off the shelf.

A WORD FROM THE SALT BOX

The recipes in this book are made using Diamond kosher salt. Diamond is a common and reasonably priced brand here in the United States (it's the one that comes in the red-and-white box).

Why do I want you to know? I've used Diamond kosher salt throughout my cooking life (and no, I'm not being paid for the mention); my parents seemed to favor it, and we always had a box in the pantry. It's cheap, found in most any grocery store, and easy to use. It dissolves easily into sauces and batters, tastes clear and salty, and plays better in recipes than the iodized table salt that fills nearly every saltshaker in America. But it wasn't until I read Samin Nosrat's masterful opus, *Salt, Fat, Acid, Heat,* that I realized not all kosher salts are created equal.

Having used Diamond my whole life, I had no idea that Morton's salt is totally different; Diamond's large-flake salt is light and crunchy, with more volume than dense Morton flakes and other chunky natural salts. The same measure of Diamond salt is less salty than Morton's, and switching out brands of salt can result in saltier recipes, if that matters to you.

Should you switch salts for this book, then? Salt *is* essential to cooking. Yet Diamond kosher salt is very reasonable at under three dollars for a 2-pound box, and it is common in most grocery stores. If you're determined to finish that box of Morton's first, go a little lighter with the salt in the dressing recipes, taste as you go, and finish the recipe with a crumb or two more if necessary. If you prefer to use sea salt, cut the salt by half, see how it works, then adjust accordingly. Thanks for reading my salt rant!

DIY MICROGREENS
A Partial Guide

Cute and crunchy, microgreens pack a ton of nutrition and flavor but often demand high prices or are just impossible to find stocked between the iceberg lettuce and bagged baby spinach. Fortunately, small-scale "harvest" microgreens are simple to grow at home and highly rewarding sources of greenery in salads throughout the year.

What exactly do I mean by microgreens? According to the urban hydroponic gardeners at Farm.One in New York City, microgreens are not sprouts (which are just the first tiny stem from a seed), but larger, slightly older babies with cotyledon leaves, the first set of leaves a young plant will grow before producing true adult leaves for the rest of its life.

I use the term *microgreen* to refer to both the young "baby leaves" plant and slightly older greens that feature their first tiny "adult" leaves. Basically tiny baby plants. Yes, you can eat these babies and still be vegan.

Traditional sprouts grown in jars, of both seeds and beans, are something I rarely cultivate at home. They require a high degree of maintenance, including rinsing several times a day to keep them moist and fresh. I rarely buy sprouts; improperly grown commercial sprouts have a highly documented track record of harboring *E. coli* and nasty bacteria, so I opt for tastier, prettier microgreens.

After some experimentation, I found that microgreens are the most forgiving, more flavorful, and relatively easy for those with less-than-green thumbs. This is my no-tech method for no-fuss sprouts.

YOU'LL NEED:

- A shallow dish or pan, no larger than 10 inches in diameter and no deeper than 2½ inches. My usual growing dish is a 10-inch round Pyrex pie plate.

- Coconut coir, a soil-like growing material made from the shells and fibers of coconuts. It's cheap and plentiful in the gardening section of big-box hardware stores. Lightweight and ultra-absorbent, one compact brick when rehydrated with water will expand to a vast amount of coir that will last you ten or more plantings.

- Spouting seeds! Do not use seeds intended for planting directly in the soil for veggie gardens, as these have been specially treated with chemicals to prevent molding. Organic spouting seeds are usually available and can be purchased by the pound or half pound (don't worry, you'll use a lot of them per batch). There are so many to choose from: broccoli, alfalfa, arugula, red kale, cabbage, radishes, and so on. When in doubt, go for a "salad mix" blend of seeds; I love seed blends for purple sprouts with purple cabbage, red kale, purple broccoli, beets, and so on.

- A spray bottle of water. The pros will tell you to use purified water, but any drinking water should do.

START YOUR SPROUT GARDENS:

- Rehydrate the coconut coir. Follow the package directions, but you'll likely only need a scant amount, as coconut coir expands to an impossible size (eight or ten times more).

- Sprinkle just under 2 inches of moistened coir into the dish. Then sprinkle an even layer of seeds over the coir.

- Spray a fine mist of water over the seeds. Cover the top of the plate snugly with plastic wrap; I hate single-use plastic wrap, but it works for odd-shaped dishes, and I reuse the same plastic as many times as possible. If you discover you love growing microgreens, consider investing in a container designed for sprouting that comes with a clear hard plastic lid.

- Now, set the plate someplace out of direct sunlight. Until the sprouts have grown into microgreens large enough to stand upright, direct sunlight is not required. Watch your first sprouts for the next 3 days or so. The warmer their environment, the faster the seeds will sprout. Don't put them on top of the radiator (too much heat), but do move the cereal boxes over on top of the fridge (just a tad warmer than everywhere else) and make some space for your seedbed.

- Check your seedbed on occasion, maybe in the morning or the afternoon over the next few days. If it seems too wet, poke a hole or two in the plastic wrap to release a little condensation. If you don't see white stems in 3 days, or the seeds start to get moldy, start over.

- Once the white baby stems are visible and the seeds have started to straighten up a bit, it's time to move them to a windowsill that gets as much daylight as possible. If it's drafty and cold, you may want to leave the plastic wrap, very loosely attached, to help contain some moisture. But if it's warm, you can remove the wrap and save it for the next round of seeds.

- Every day, check the soil and mist your sprouts with water if the soil looks dry. In about 8 to 10 days, the microgreens should have green (or purple) healthy-looking early leaves. Trim them by the palmful with scissors, rinse, pat dry, and eat right away. Compost the used coir bed and start again!

For a really in-depth exploration of how to grow vigorously healthy and bountiful greens, or in his words, "soil sprouts," check out *Year-Round Indoor Salad Gardening* by Peter Burke (from Chelsea Green Publishing). It's an intensely nerdy read about his cheap and practical system for growing a lot of large microgreens, using a little bit of dirt and small containers you already own. A solid system to follow, especially if you dream of growing your own hearty, juicy sunflower seed sprouts, which are like the asparagus of sprouts (or if you hate asparagus, insert your other favorite sweet substantial stalk veggie). Peter will school you in far greater depth than I can about how to grow an astounding amount of salad on your windowsill.

If you can't be bothered and want an attractive houseplant-style, "just add water" approach, try out the Hama hydroponic seed mat (hamama.cc). If "hydroponics" in your home sends you sweating about installing a system of tubes and pumps and pipes in your living room, this is a no-tech, pre-seeded mat that sits in a nice-looking, water-once tray. Ten or so days later, you will have little clusters of petite greens to snip and eat. Not enough to fill a salad bowl, but great for garnishing and adding a little zing to avocado toast. It costs more than really DIYing it with seeds and dirt, but it's as easy and neat as homegrown can be.

In New York City and want to see hydroponic microgreens and fancy restaurant baby plants grown by the masters? Schedule a visit or a class at Farm.One (farm.one); nestled deep inside the Institute of Culinary Education in downtown Manhattan, the nice folks there will show you a tiny microbiome far away from natural sunlight that produces a dazzling array of uncommon herbs and edible flowers, all cultivated in a room the size of a New York City master bedroom / suburban walk-in closet. Everybody asks for a taste of the toothache plant flower, but those in the know ask to nibble on baby mustard greens or minty nepitella blossoms.

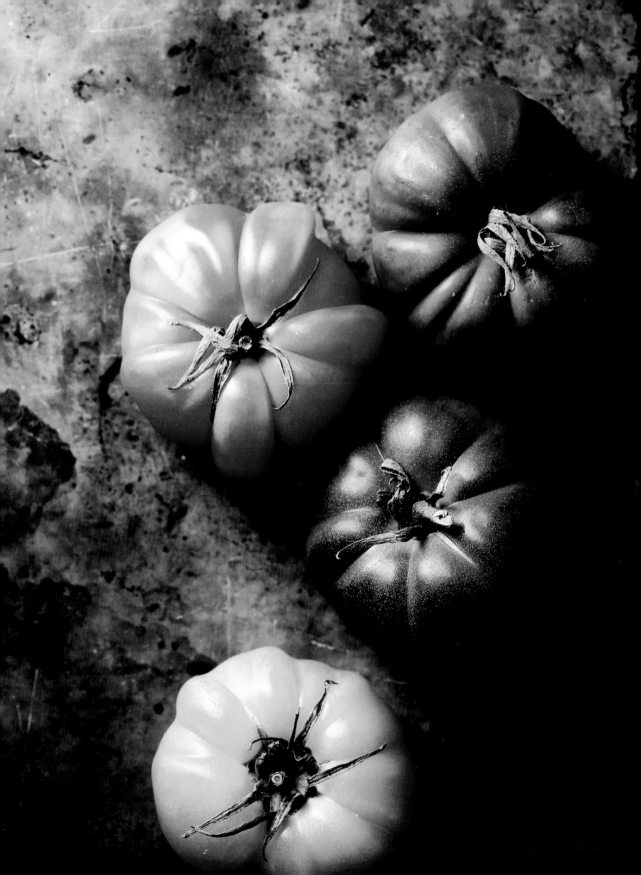

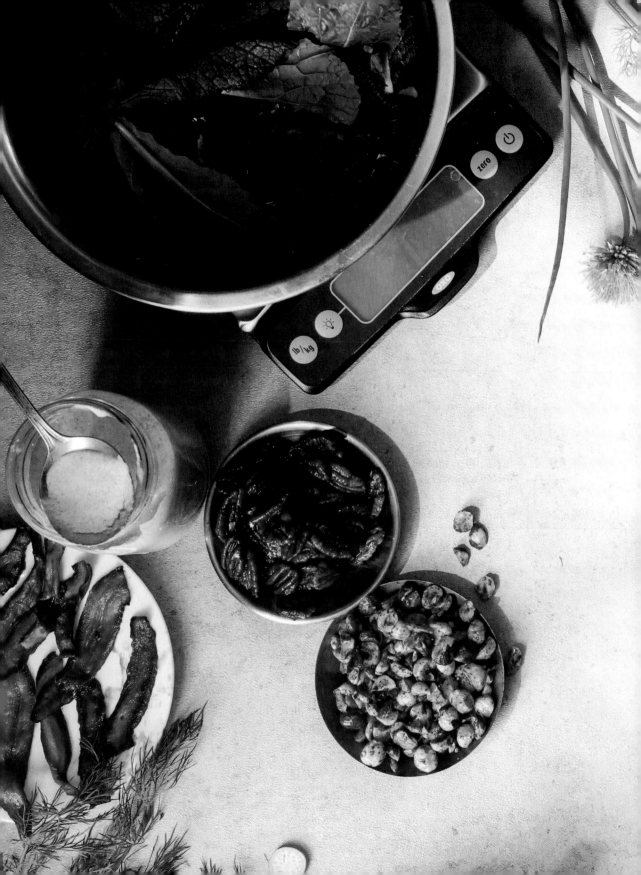

SALADS FOR NERDS
How to Make Salad with a Scale

While working at a start-up recently, I got to chatting with one of the engineers about my ongoing salad recipe research and development. He asked, "Why doesn't anyone make salad with a scale?" This could be the ultimate fast and no-hassle salad: a kitchen scale (preferably a digital one for one-button ease) can measure the ideal amount of each ingredient for a consistent serving of salad every time. If the idea of consistently measured salad sounds strange to you, recall that salad bars across the country rely on weighing our salads. Just imagine how many unplanned twenty-three-dollar lunchtime salads you could avoid each week if a scale were an option while *building* the salad!

Once you have a few toppings, some freshly washed veggies, and a homemade dressing stashed in the fridge, making a big salad with the help of your scale makes the salad assembling process simple and speedy. Below is an "un-recipe," a loose guide to assembling a big, leafy green salad packed with toppings, dressings, and additional fresh veggies. This makes a big salad, but reduce the amount of veggies by roughly half or so for smaller appetites.

---

4 to 5 ounces leafy greens or hearty greens, washed, spun dry, torn into bite-sized pieces

3 to 4 ounces cooked pasta, grains, or potato

2 to 3 ounces diced tofu/tempeh, seitan, chickpeas, salad lentils, or other legumes

2 ounces hearty vegetables: shredded cabbage, thinly

sliced red onions, shredded carrots, diced broccoli/cauliflower, etc.

1 to 2 ounces croutons or roasted nut toppings

1 to 2 ounces juicy vegetables or fruits: tomatoes, cucumber, grapes, or diced/chopped fruit

½ to 1 ounce freshly made vinaigrette or creamy dressing

Get a kitchen scale. Digital scales make this nearly effortless, but analog scales can work if you're comfortable resetting the weight manually.

Place the mixing bowl on the scale; tare (set to zero) the scale.

Add each ingredient or component (already made dressing/toppings) as listed, per the weight amounts at left, then hit tare to reset the weight after each ingredient.

When you're done, use tongs to toss everything together.

Transfer your precision salad to a serving bowl (or not—just eat out of the mixing bowl!) and garnish with anything else you want more of. An extra dash of dressing is a solid win for enjoying more flavor with your salad.

STASH THAT SALAD

Salads and salad ingredients should be eaten and cooked with as soon as possible. There are exceptions (e.g., croutons, some toppings, and most dressings). I've made note in each recipe as to a general time frame of when they simply just taste best, but in case you need the notes of the how and when to eat salad ingredients, here's a general list. Produce from the garden or farmers' market tends to be fresher, and lasts a bit longer, than the average supermarket vegetable. Your mileage may vary!

UNWASHED GREENS, FRESH HERBS, BERRIES, TENDER VEGGIES (PEA SHOOTS, ETC.):

- Store loosely covered in the veggie bin of the fridge.

- Use within a week, or less/more depending on freshness.

UNWASHED, UNSLICED, FIRM VEGETABLES AND FRUITS (EGGPLANTS, CAULIFLOWER, CARROTS, RIPENING PEACHES, ETC.):

- Store wrapped and/or covered in the veggie bin of the fridge.

- Use within 8 to 10 days, or less/more depending on freshness.

POTATOES, ONIONS, GARLIC, APPLES:

- Store in a cool, dark, dry cabinet and use within 2 weeks.

WASHED, DRIED GREENS AND TENDER VEGGIES; SLICED, FIRM VEGETABLES:

- Store tightly covered in the veggie bin of the fridge.

- Use within 3 to 5 days, or less/more depending on freshness.

- Store tightly covered in a cool, dark, dry place.

- Use within 2 weeks, or less/more depending on humidity levels in the kitchen or pantry.

DRESSINGS, MARINADES, SAUCES, AND MARINATING ITEMS; COOKED MOIST TOPPINGS (TOFU, ROASTED VEGETABLES); COOKED GRAINS / PASTA, SOUP:

- Keep chilled and tightly covered in the fridge.

- Use or prepare within 1 to 3 days.

FULLY DRESSED AND READY-TO-GO SALAD:

- Eat immediately! If you must, keep covered and chilled and eat within 2 to 6 hours.

TO THE GLUTEN-FREE, NUT-FREE, SOY-FREE SALAD ENTHUSIAST

As recipes go, almost all the recipes in this book can be made free of gluten, nuts, and soy with a few substitutions. Here are some general guidelines for changing recipes.

GLUTEN-FREE

Most of these recipes are gluten-free. For obviously bready ones (croutons), use your favorite **gluten-free bread.** For farro or bulgur, swap in **quinoa.**

NUT-FREE

The hemp- and sunflower-based dressings use a small amount of almond milk. Use your favorite unflavored type, preferably **unsweetened hemp, rice,** or **oat milk.** Soy milk can also be used, but it may transform the consistency of the dressing into a thick mayonnaise-like spread. Not bad, just different. Experiment and see what works for you.

SOY-FREE

Use seitan made without soy sauce (make your own using coconut aminos, page 81) or beans in place of soy foods. Try **coconut aminos** in place of soy sauce and tamari. In place of white miso (soy based), use **chickpea miso** (available in health food stores).

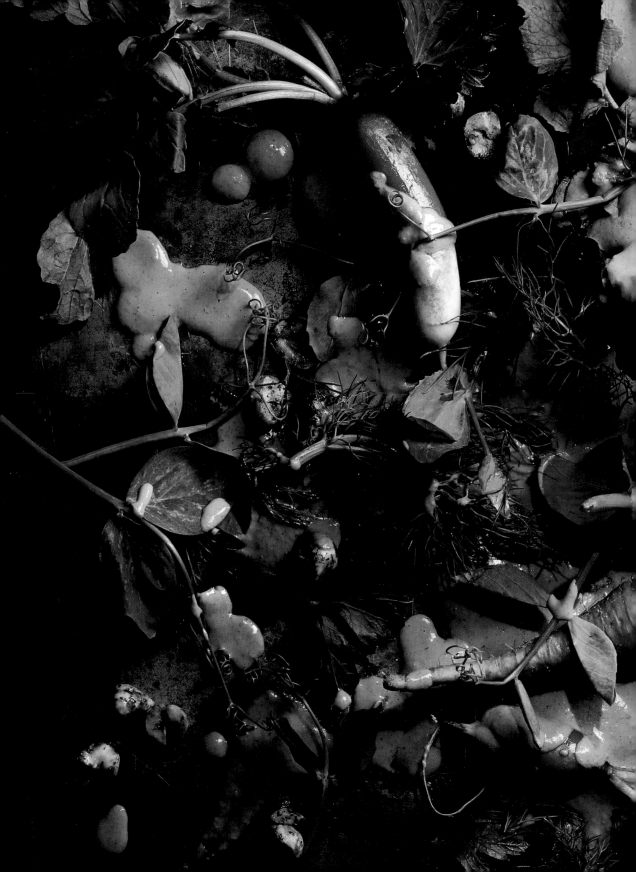

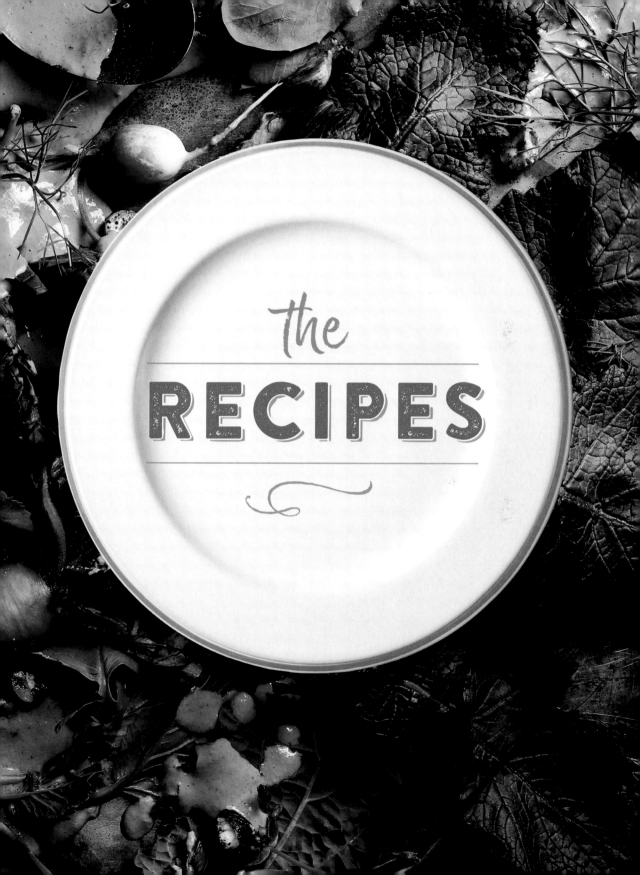

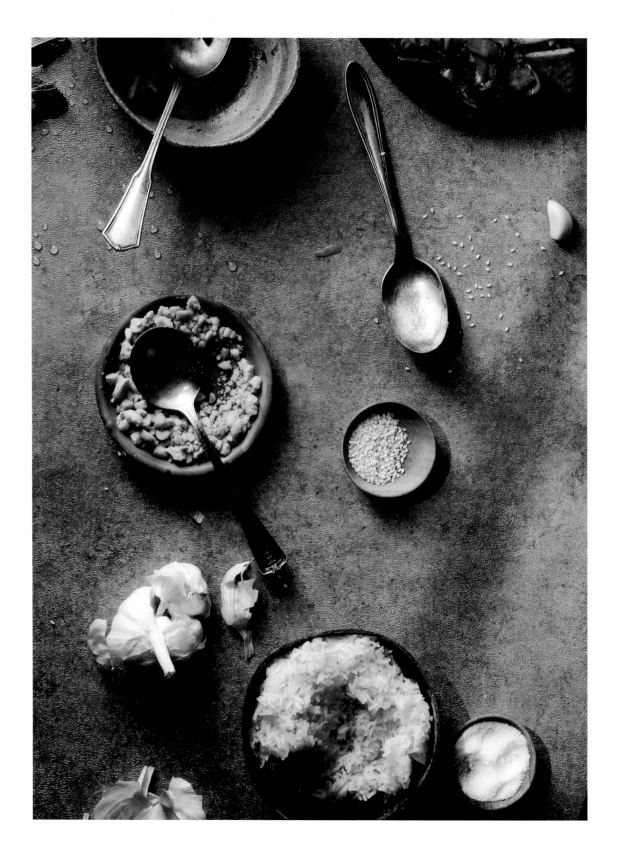

DRESSINGS and TOPPINGS

~

Smartly Dressed Salads

DRESSINGS

Homemade dressing and hearty toppings are what set apart a thoughtfully composed salad from a pile of vegetables topped with store-bought salad glue (I have strong opinions about salad dressing). Creating your own dressings, roasted root bacon, seasoned roasted nuts, or playfully flavored baked tofu takes more effort than ordering takeout, but it's time well spent. Less junky convenience food, fewer plastic takeout containers, and more healthful fresh ingredients. Salad can be simple, but it never should be boring!

TIPS FOR SMARTLY DRESSED SALAD

Salad dressing—the most appropriate, descriptive name for a food. Without it, a salad is naked, just a pile of leaves and perhaps a few cubes of old bread.

If there's one thing I hope you gain from this book, it's that making your own dressing is a pleasure. Even store-bought dressings made with organic ingredients will never taste as clean and fresh as a freshly made batch of homemade dressing. Making really delicious homemade dressings is easy and so rewarding that you'll want to throw off the shackles of bottled salad dressing forever!

Layered Dressings

Occasionally, I will recommend tossing a small amount of a simple oil-acid-salt vinaigrette to leafy greens or produce before dressing the final salad with a creamy dressing.

This layering of dressings is helpful; it opens up the biggest flavors from the ingredients and renders chewy leaves (kale, collards, etc.) tender. In many of my hearty salads with roasted ingredients, you'll find that I prefer a simple vinaigrette to season the leaves, then pass around richer, thicker dressings to spoon on top.

The Dressing Pantry Dream Team

Dream teams are assembled to fight supervillains and take down the system or to craft the perfect metal album. Those teams are hard to put together and take a lot of people, but you can assemble a dream team of pantry-friendly dressing ingredients in one simple shopping trip. Stocking a shelf with these and making a fresh batch of vinaigrette or a generous portion of creamy dressing won't be a chore but a step you'll look forward to for making great meals. See ***The Salad Pantry: Everything but the Veggies*** (page 11) for a full shopping list; the dressing essentials I always have on hand are:

- Extra-virgin olive oil: a large, economical bottle for gentle cooking and a higher-quality one for dressings and drizzling after cooking.

- Grape-seed oil: neutral tasting, light textured, easy to use, and relatively healthy. Safflower and sunflower oils are good stand-ins for grape-seed oil.

- White wine vinegar, red wine vinegar, apple cider, and balsamic vinegar: I don't use regular household white vinegar, which tends to be too harsh for salads (but always great for cleaning the kitchen when you're done).

- Dijon mustard and mustard powder: More than just flavor, mustards are sublime emulsifiers for stable, smooth vinaigrettes.

- Kosher salt, Diamond brand: If you skipped my rant about salt, shame on you. We'll still be friends if you go read it now (page 13).

- Lemons, limes, shallots, garlic: essential seasonings, fresh but long-lasting produce that can last a week or longer properly stored (in a cool, dry, dark place).

HOW TO GET DRESSED

Just as you wouldn't put on a T-shirt after styling your hair or struggle to fit tube socks under a pair of skinny jeans, there are better ways to get your beautiful homemade salad dressing into a salad. Better-looking salads really *do* taste better too!

DON'T pour all the dressing over dry, leafy salad ingredients, then skip away from your meal for hours. Dress and eat pronto. Overnight salad isn't as charming as overnight oats.

DO drizzle a tablespoon of dressing over the firm, juicy elements of the salad first. Gently stir to coat. With generously portioned creamy dressings, it's better to coat the salad with a spoonful or two, then pass around the rest and let eaters (or just you) drizzle on dressing over assembled salad.

$\mathcal{DON'T}$ slap it all down in one big messy pile. It's okay if it's just you, in old baggy-knees leggings and a comfy T-shirt, eating salad directly out of the salad spinner on occasion. But it's nice to spend a few minutes building a beautiful salad to share with others. Or even if just feeding yourself.

$\mathcal{DO}$ build your salad upward, instead of outward and flat. Stacking salad leaves, toppings, and dressing in layers builds height and excitement to even the simplest concoctions. As you can see by the photos in this book, salads can be sculpted on not just dinner plates but platters, flat plates, even baking trays to dish up salad for a crowd!

Tip

MAIN SQUEEZES

While freshly squeezed lemon and citrus juice is best, there are some exceptions. Bottled can be convenient, and organic, not-from-concentrate lemon and lime juices can be great; use 100 percent juice, in glass bottles, and taste like real fruit juice. Read your citrus juice bottle labels, and when in doubt, use fresh produce. Avoid the plastic lemon- or lime-shaped bottles of citrus "juice": It's just more plastic that will end up in the wastestream, and most often the stuff in them is a composite of juice, water, and citrus oil that does not taste like good-quality citrus juice.

CREAMY DRESSINGS SO MANY WAYS

Vegan dressings have an exciting variety of ways to get that dairy-free creaminess: puréed soaked nuts and seeds, nut milks, coconut milk, and soy products. Store the following pantry items in your fridge for optimal freshness and many creamy dressings to come:

Unroasted "raw" cashew pieces. Cheaper than whole cashews. Sometimes mislabeled *raw* (all cashews must be minimally processed to remove naturally occurring toxins), unroasted cashews have a mellow, creamy, slightly sweet flavor.

Raw sunflower seeds, sliced or slivered almonds (blanched or unpeeled), shelled hemp seeds, sesame seeds, chia seeds, coconut milk, and sesame tahini.

Go for organic when possible, and store nuts in the fridge during warm months to keep them fresh longer. Write the date on a newly purchased package of nuts and use within 4 months for the best flavor and freshness (rancid nuts and seeds can easily mess up the flavor of a creamy dressing—not the nutty kind of surprise you want to have).

THE ZEN OF HEMP DRESSING

Shelled hemp seeds—also called *hemp hearts*—are nutritious, somewhat soft, easy-to-digest seeds loaded with healthy fatty acids. They won't get you high, but they make a killer creamy dressing.

These hemp-based dressings are prepared similarly to a mayonnaise, by whipping together the emulsifier ingredient (in this vegan instance, hemp seeds blended with almond milk) with oil to create the creamy base. After the base has been crafted, we'll flavor it with the perfect balance of acid, aromatics, herbs, spices, and, of course, salt! Use the Caesar or ranch dressing as a core recipe, one that can be shaped and adjusted to create a wide range of flavorful, creamy dressings.

Your choice of nondairy milk also makes a difference with hemp and other creamy dressings. Almond milk is my favorite smooth, creamy dressing ready to pour. For dressings, always use unsweetened, unflavored almond milk or your favorite nut- or seed-based milk. Soy milk will quickly create a mayonnaise style— probably not ideal for pouring onto salad. The exception? Thick, whipped soy milk dressings are very spreadable (great for sandwiches), and the perfect consistency for Chickpea Pickle Collard Wraps (page 170). Try a batch one day with almond milk, and then soy milk the next time, and appreciate the great differences a different plant milk can make!

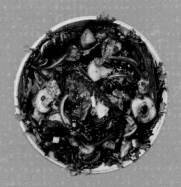

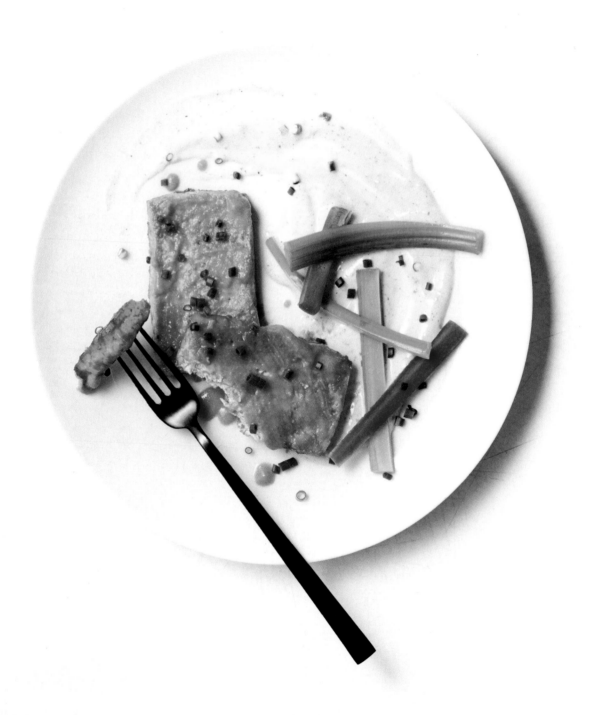

HEMP SEED CAESAR DRESSING

Makes about ¾ cup

DELICIOUS ON:

Forever Kale Caesar with Cheesy, Crispy Croutons (page 163)

Chickpea Pickle Collard Wraps (page 170)

Any big, leafy salad with lots of crunchy greens

3 tablespoons shelled hemp seeds

¼ cup unsweetened plain almond milk or nut-free plain vegan milk

½ cup olive oil

2 tablespoons capers, drained (save the brine, to season the dressing later)

2 tablespoons nutritional yeast

2 to 3 garlic cloves, peeled

1 tablespoon white wine vinegar

1 tablespoon lemon juice

2 teaspoons Dijon mustard

1 teaspoon kosher salt

When imagining the ideal salad, Caesar salad has captured our collective heart and stomach. Or more specifically, that briny-garlicky-fatty-cheesy dressing that so beautifully grabs onto leafy greens and toasted bread. The hemp seed base provides the slightly grainy, fatty bits of seeds reminiscent of grated Parmesan. Along with capers for the required anchovy-like brine, the traditional Caesar ingredients of lemon juice, wine vinegar, and plenty of olive oil burst through. It's the dressing code that, once cracked, opens up variations that fit into any role and can dress any green—and even in some instances flavors other salad-worthy garnishes (see Caesar Walnuts, page 123).

Blend together the hemp seeds and the almond milk for 30 seconds. Slowly stream in the oil into the blender jar and pulse until the dressing is thick and silky. The dressing base is ready but rather plain, so it's now time to add the elements of flavor. Add the capers, nutritional yeast, garlic, white wine vinegar, lemon juice, mustard, and salt and blend for 30 seconds or more until evenly blended.

Taste the dressing; if it needs a little more salt, add a pinch of kosher salt or drizzle in a teaspoon or two of caper brine; if it tastes a little flat, add a teaspoon of lemon juice. Use right away or, if possible, chill for 30 minutes and allow the flavors to meld. This dressing tastes best if used within a day of making.

HEMP SEED TARRAGON DIJON DRESSING

Makes 1 cup

DELICIOUS ON:

Roasted Niçoise Salad (page 188)

The Bright and Spicy Spring Asparagus Salad (page 151)

Romaine and butter lettuce / dandelion greens / spring radishes / snap peas / chilled cooked potatoes

3 tablespoons shelled hemp seeds

¼ cup unsweetened plain almond milk or nut-free plain vegan milk

½ cup extra-virgin olive oil

1 small shallot, peeled and chopped

2 tablespoons lemon juice

1 tablespoon white wine vinegar

2 tablespoons Dijon mustard

1 teaspoon kosher salt

1 tablespoon chopped fresh tarragon or 1 teaspoon dried tarragon

This hardworking hemp seed and almond milk dressing is *the* perfect garnish for Roasted Niçoise Salad, any salad with potatoes, or just a pile of crisp greens and perfectly ripe tomatoes.

In a blender, pulse together the hemp seeds and the almond milk for 30 seconds. Slowly stream in the oil and pulse until the dressing is thick and silky. Add the shallot, lemon juice, vinegar, mustard, and salt and blend for another 30 seconds until smooth. Add the tarragon to the dressing and pulse for 1 to 2 seconds.

Taste the dressing; if it needs a little more salt, add a pinch of kosher salt or drizzle in a teaspoon or less of vinegar. Use right away or, if possible, chill for 30 minutes and allow the flavors to meld. This dressing tastes best if used within a day of making.

CREAMY ITALIAN HEMP DRESSING

Makes 1 cup

DELICIOUS ON:

The Juicy Grilled Summer Days Peach Salad (page 155)

Sriracha Ranch Salad Party (instead of Sriracha Cilantro Ranch Dressing) (page 165)

Ruffled kale / steamed broccoli / roasted cauliflower / steamed sweet potatoes

3 tablespoons shelled hemp seeds

¼ cup unsweetened plain almond milk or nut-free plain vegan milk

½ cup mild-tasting olive oil

2 tablespoons lemon juice

1 tablespoon red wine vinegar

2 garlic cloves, peeled

1 teaspoon kosher salt

1 tablespoon off-the-shelf Italian seasoning dried herb blend

¼ teaspoon red pepper flakes

Beloved in strip mall pizza-pasta parlors everywhere, the concoction called "creamy Italian" dressing can be truly transformative when prepared from scratch. And what better way to embrace it than using off-the-shelf Italian herb seasoning, the American mashup of dried basil, oregano, and marjoram with the occasional dash of thyme, sage, or parsley. It's ranch dressing reborn in an Italian restaurant spiked with pizza herbs and olive oil. But the flavors are beyond ordinary.

In a blender, pulse together the hemp seeds and the almond milk for 30 seconds. Slowly stream in the oil and pulse until the dressing is thick and silky. Add the remaining ingredients and blend for another 30 seconds until evenly blended.

Taste the dressing; if it needs a little more salt, add a pinch of kosher salt, or if it tastes a little flat, add a few drops of lemon juice. If possible, chill for 30 minutes and allow the flavors to meld. Use within 3 days for the best flavor.

Tip

No Italian seasoning? Use 1 teaspoon oregano, 1 teaspoon dried basil, ½ teaspoon dried marjoram, ½ teaspoon dried rosemary, ½ teaspoon dried thyme, and a pinch of powdered sage.

HORSERADISH HEMP DRESSING

Makes 1 cup

THIS IS REALLY TASTY ON:

Blackened Tempeh Reuben Salad (page 179)

Blanched green beans / roasted carrots / chopped snap peas /
red onion / red potatoes / cauliflower

3 tablespoons shelled hemp seeds

¼ cup unsweetened plain almond milk or nut-free plain vegan milk

½ cup olive oil

2 tablespoons red wine vinegar

1 tablespoon tomato paste

1 tablespoon lemon juice

1 garlic clove, minced

1 teaspoon kosher salt

1 teaspoon hot paprika or 1 teaspoon paprika plus ¼ teaspoon cayenne pepper

1 tablespoon grated horseradish or prepared horseradish

¼ cup minced white onion

This is Russian dressing, the spicy sibling of Thousand Island, reborn with a hemp seed base and pumped up with horseradish. Minced white onion adds texture, tomato paste in place of sugary ketchup provides the essential hint of tomato, and there is a spicy double kick from hot paprika and prepared horseradish.

In a blender, pulse together the hemp seeds and the almond milk for 30 seconds. Slowly stream in the oil and pulse until the dressing is thick and silky. Add in the remaining ingredients and blend for another 30 seconds until evenly blended.

Taste the dressing; if it needs a little more salt, add a pinch of kosher salt, or if it tastes a little flat, add a few drops of lemon juice. If possible, chill for 30 minutes and allow the flavors to meld. Use within 3 days for the best flavor.

THE WAY OF
SUNFLOWER SEED DRESSINGS

In my previous salad book, *Salad Samurai*, all my rich, creamy dressings were made with a base of soaked, unroasted cashews. Cashews are still essential for so many versatile, dairy-like dressings and sauces, but a few years and many requests for nut-free dressings later, I've leaned on sunflower seeds as a stand-in for cashews for creating that satisfying dairy-like richness.

Besides not being a nut (a relief for those with nut allergies), sunflower seeds are common and cheap. And if you fancy the idea of growing your own cashews and live hundreds of miles from the tropics (cashew trees are evergreens that grow only in tropical zones), you're outta luck. But hardy, fast-growing sunflower seeds flourish in temperate climates and are a great addition to any salad garden.

This is a drizzling-style dressing, meaning it's substantial and creamy yet just loose enough to pour over greens or as a dipping sauce. Just like cashew-based dressings, the rules for using sunflower seeds remain the same: Seeds must be unroasted, unsalted, and as fresh as possible. Fresh sunflower seeds taste mild and slightly sweet.

Sunflower seeds must be soaked in cold water for at least an hour, or covered and in the fridge overnight. Pour off the soaking water, rinse plumped seeds with cold water, and blend soaked seeds with enough liquid to create the creamy dressing base. For best results, use the most powerful blender you can get (Blendtec, Vitamix, Ninja) for the smoothest dressings.

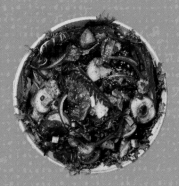

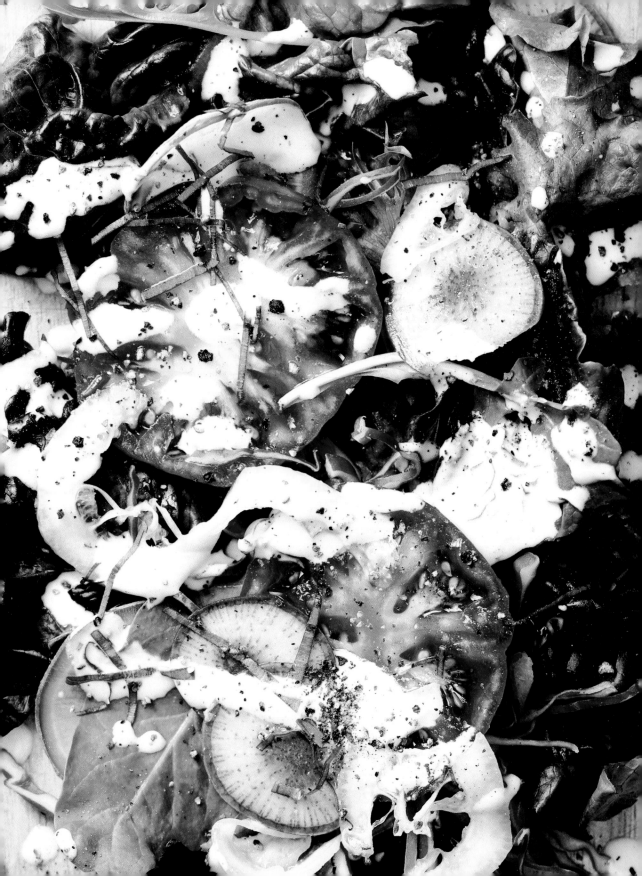

SUNFLOWER RANCH DRESSING

Makes 1⅓ cups

TRY IT SPOONED OVER:

Charred Broccoli, Potato, and Root Bacon Salad (page 229)

The Big Crunchy Autumn Vibes Salad (page 159)

Roasted Niçoise Salad (a free-form Niçoise Salad) (page 188)

Any crunchy lettuce / tomatoes / cucumbers / chickpeas

½ cup raw sunflower seeds, soaked for 1 hour minimum, or overnight

½ cup unsweetened plain almond milk, cashew milk, or your choice nut-free vegan milk

1 tablespoon lemon juice

1 tablespoon white wine vinegar

1 big fat garlic clove, peeled

1 teaspoon dried onion flakes or ½ teaspoon onion powder

1 teaspoon kosher salt

Several generous twists of black pepper

3 tablespoons grape-seed oil or mild-tasting olive oil

1 tablespoon minced fresh or 1 teaspoon dried parsley

1 tablespoon minced fresh or 1 teaspoon dried dill

Ranch dressing, cool, creamy, flecked with fresh herbs, is as versatile as a creamy dressing can be. Made completely vegan and with the combination of sunflower seeds and nut milk (or oat or coconut beverage if you're avoiding nuts), this dressing is ready to be poured all over greens or veggies, or even used as a dip for tofu nuggets.

I prefer a thinner dressing for pouring, but if you prefer a thicker dressing (as did my testers), reduce the vegan milk to ⅓ cup. Along with any hemp seed dressings, this is my go-to salad sauce.

Drain the sunflower seeds. In a blender, blend everything except the oil and herbs into a smooth, creamy mixture. Scrape down the sides of the blender jar several times with a rubber spatula and keep blending until as smooth as possible, about 2 to 3 minutes.

Continued

Drizzle in the oil a little at a time, pulsing until the mixture is smooth and emulsified. If a thinner texture is desired, pulse in a tablespoon of water at a time until the desired texture is reached. Add the fresh or dried herbs and pulse once or twice to combine. Store in a tightly covered container in the fridge and use within 2 days for the best flavor.

Tip

This dressing is flavorful as it is, but you can push it further with:

- 1 teaspoon organic sugar or agave nectar (a bit of sweetness helps pull together the flavors)
- ½ teaspoon celery seed
- ¼ cup minced chives

SUN AND SEA SUNFLOWER CAESAR DRESSING

Makes about 1 cup

½ cup raw sunflower seeds, soaked for 2 hours or overnight

½ cup unsweetened plain almond milk, cashew milk, or your choice nut-free vegan milk

1 heaping tablespoon nutritional yeast

6 Kalamata olives, pits removed

1 tablespoon olive brine

2 teaspoons rice vinegar

2 teaspoons white miso

2 garlic cloves, peeled

2 teaspoons powdered seaweed (arame, kelp, nori, etc.)

Big pinch sea salt

Several generous twists of black pepper

¼ cup mild olive oil

One can never have too many Caesar dressings! This sunflower-based dressing is a cost-effective alternative to the hemp Caesar. For the essential briny flavor, instead of capers, this dressing uses Kalamata olives—the enduringly favorite purple-black Greek olive with juicy flesh—and a dash of dried seaweed adds a bit of oceanic flavor. Arame, a reddish edible seaweed that is a health food store staple and commonly available in an easy-to-use powder, is my favorite, along with powdered kelp or, if you can find it, powdered nori.

Drain the sunflower seeds. Blend everything except the oil into a smooth, creamy mixture. Scrape down the sides of the blender jar several times with a rubber spatula.

Drizzle in the oil a little at a time, pulsing until the mixture is smooth and emulsified. If a thinner texture is desired, pulse in a tablespoon of water at a time until the desired texture is reached. Taste the dressing and adjust the seasoning by adding a teaspoon or more of olive brine or nutritional yeast as desired. Store in a tightly covered container in the fridge and use within 2 days for the best flavor.

SRIRACHA CILANTRO RANCH DRESSING

Makes about 1 cup

½ cup raw sunflower seeds, soaked for 2 hours or overnight

½ cup unsweetened plain almond milk, cashew milk, or your choice nut-free vegan milk

2 tablespoons freshly squeezed lime juice

1 tablespoon rice vinegar

1 big fat garlic clove, peeled

1 teaspoon kosher salt

Several generous twists of freshly ground black pepper

¼ cup grape-seed oil or mild-tasting olive oil

2 tablespoons chopped cilantro, leaves and tender stems

2 tablespoons sriracha hot sauce or sambal oelek paste, or more to taste

Perhaps one of the most important celebrity marriages of the century is the union of cool ranch dressing and beloved and enduring hot and garlicky sriracha chile sauce. Don't miss out on this one; it's one of my top picks for creamy dressing to go with most anything. The Southeast Asian flavors (cilantro, lime, hot chile garlic) go great drizzled on American eats such as veggie burgers and pizza. In a pinch, sambal oelek, the increasingly popular Indonesian condiment of crushed whole red chiles, is also great in this exciting dressing.

Drain the sunflower seeds. Blend everything except the oil, cilantro, and sriracha into a smooth, creamy mixture, for at least 2 to 3 minutes. Scrape down the sides of the blender jar several times with a rubber spatula during the blending process.

Drizzle in the oil a little at a time, pulsing until the mixture is smooth and emulsified. If a thinner texture is desired, pulse in a tablespoon of water at a time until the desired texture is reached. Add the cilantro and the sriracha and pulse a few times to blend. Store in a tightly covered container in the fridge and use within 2 days for the best flavor.

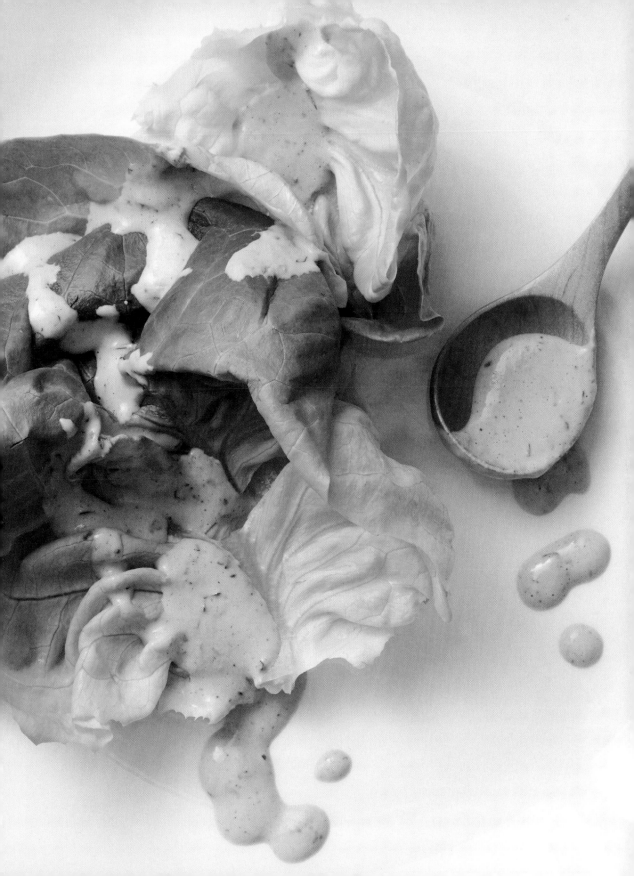

TAHINI-BASED CREAMY DRESSINGS

Creamy, velvety, naturally packed with buttery flavors, tahini has been loved for years as a base for killer vegan dressings. It's hard to go wrong with tahini in the mix! It's also the base for my favorite extra-fatty take on retro-delicious French dressing.

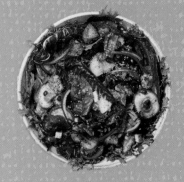

TAHINI MAYO

Makes 1½ cups

THIS IS REALLY TASTY ON:

Any avocado toast, but especially Avocado and Black Bean Salad
on Cornbread Toast (page 243)

Mustard Greens Tabbouleh with Almonds and Roasted Chickpeas
(page 222)

Lazy Seitan Gyro Spinach Salad (page 204)

¼ cup freshly
squeezed lemon
juice

1 teaspoon
agave nectar

1 teaspoon
mustard powder

1 teaspoon
kosher salt

½ cup sesame
tahini

¼ cup mild olive oil
or grape-seed oil

Velvety and buttery, this hearty mayo-like spread, a kind of whipped sesame tahini, works great with so many other ingredients. What started out as a tahini dressing turned into a thick spread too good to turn away from, but if you're partial to tahini dressings, you can always increase the water to reach a consistency that suits you best. Note that if you make the recipe as is, the olive oil flavor will be very pronounced; it's delicious, but if you want something a little more neutral, substitute half or all the olive oil with mild-tasting grape-seed oil, which also provides that classic mayonnaise flavor.

Add the lemon juice, ¼ cup of water, agave nectar, mustard powder, salt, and tahini to a food processor or blender. Pulse until smooth and blended. Stream in the oil, pulsing and stopping to scrape down the sides of the bowl occasionally. The finished tahini mayo will be thick, rich, and silky. Keep chilled and use within 3 days for the best flavor.

variation

TAHINI DRESSING

For a smooth and easy-to-pour dressing, increase the water to up to ½ cup. Taste and add more salt or even a teaspoon or two more oil to balance out the flavors.

TURMERIC TAHINI MISO SAUCE

Makes 1½ cups

TRY THIS WITH:

Protein-Packed Salad for Breakfast (page 191)

Kabocha and Black Rice Salad (page 195)

Green Again Soup with Tahini Miso Slaw (page 253)

Shredded cabbage / radishes / cauliflower / broccoli

1½ teaspoons turmeric powder

½ teaspoon ground ginger

½ teaspoon ground black pepper

¼ teaspoon ground cardamom

2 tablespoons freshly squeezed lemon juice

⅓ cup sesame tahini

2 tablespoons white miso

¼ teaspoon kosher salt, or to taste

Tahini and miso, whisked together with enough water to form a smooth and silky dressing, have comprised my go-to salad and vegetable sauce for decades. This health-guru version is spiked with turmeric for an Instagram-health-blogger-worthy sauce that can go on virtually everything, including, of course, salad. The most important step is simmering the turmeric powder with water (as tahini sauces always need plenty of water); don't skip this step and toss in the turmeric raw. Cooking turmeric by some accounts makes some of the antioxidants more bioavailable, and I find the flavor of simmered turmeric to be smoother and more complex than harsh-tasting raw turmeric.

In a small saucepan, combine ¾ cup of water, turmeric, ginger, black pepper, and cardamom. Over medium heat, bring to a rapid simmer, cover, reduce the heat to low, and simmer gently for about 3 minutes. Turn off the heat and cool for a minute.

Pour into a blender, add the remaining ingredients, and pulse until smooth. Scrape down the sides of the blender a few times. Taste and add a pinch more of salt or dash of lemon, if desired. Chill in a tightly covered container and use within 3 days for the best flavor.

TAHINI FRENCH DRESSING

Makes 1½ cups

THIS IS REALLY TASTY ON:

Crunchy Eggplant Parm Salad (page 207)

Sriracha Ranch Salad Party (page 165)

The Big Crunchy Autumn Vibes Salad (page 159)

Romaine lettuce / tomatoes / sweet white onion / grilled eggplant

2 tablespoons red wine vinegar

3 tablespoons tomato paste

1 tablespoon freshly squeezed lemon juice

2 tablespoons agave nectar

1 tablespoon Dijon mustard

1 garlic clove, peeled (or minced if mixing by hand)

1 teaspoon kosher salt

½ teaspoon sweet paprika

A few twists of freshly ground pepper

⅓ cup good-quality olive oil

½ cup sesame tahini

Made with tahini for an outrageously creamy and umami-loaded dressing, old-fashioned French dressing will never be the same again. August tomatoes and peak-season cucumbers demand this tangy, luscious concoction. My favorite snacking salad—ruffled kale, shreds of crisp red cabbage, half-moons of sweet white onion—reaches perfection when tossed with a few spoons of this sunset-hued dressing.

Add ¾ cup of water, red wine vinegar, tomato paste, lemon juice, agave, mustard, garlic, salt, and paprika to a blender and pulse until very smooth. Or, in a mixing bowl and a wire whisk, whisk all these ingredients together until smooth.

Stream in the oil, pulsing/whisking and stopping to scrape down the sides of the bowl occasionally. Add the tahini a spoonful at a time and only pulse enough until blended and smooth; do not overmix with a blender (if whisking by hand, mix until smooth). Chill for 20 minutes before serving for the best flavor. Like any tahini dressing, this will thicken up the longer it sits, so go ahead and whisk in a tablespoon or two of cold water to loosen it up a bit before serving.

OIL-FREE CASHEW LEMON PEPPER DRESSING

Makes 1¼ cups

TRY THIS WITH:

Charred Broccoli, Potato, and Root Bacon Salad (page 229)

Sriracha Ranch Salad Party (instead of the Sriracha Cilantro Ranch Dressing) (page 165)

Any and all big, green leafy salads!

¼ cup unroasted cashew pieces, soaked for 30 minutes and drained

½ cup unsweetened plain almond milk

3 tablespoons lemon juice

1 tablespoon white wine vinegar

1 big fat garlic clove, peeled

1 teaspoon grated lemon zest

1 teaspoon mustard powder

1 teaspoon kosher salt

1 tablespoon chia seeds (see Chia Notes, below)

2 teaspoons whole black peppercorns, cracked

I was initially resistant to the idea of a no-oil dressing, but after some experimentation, this has become one of my favorites. Creamy, tangy, and robust, it's now on regular rotation in my salad routine. The super duo of raw cashews and almond milk are unmatched for adding substance and a neutral canvas for fresh herbs and spices. Together they create a bountiful ranch-style dressing, just over a cup, perfect for drizzling over big, crunchy leafy summer salads or sturdy, leafy, cool-weather kale salad, or even just gently blanched broccoli.

Blend all the ingredients except for the chia seeds and pepper until very smooth. Keep the dressing in the blender jar and sprinkle in the seeds, stir, set aside to gel for 5 minutes. In a mortar and pestle, crush the black peppercorns into chunky grains, then add to the dressing in the blender jar. Pulse a few times to blend in the chia seeds and black pepper. Chill for 30 minutes before using to develop the flavor and texture.

PEPPERCORNS: CRACKED, GROUND, AND DUSTY

For years, cracked versus ground black pepper were the same to me (embarrassing)—anything was better than the dusty stuff from a tin can that most of us grew up identifying as "black pepper."

But there's an important difference between pepper freshly fallen out of a grinder and chunky, crunchy cracked peppercorns. Freshly ground pepper is superior to canned black pepper. But chunky hand-cracked pepper makes a statement on a salad or bathed in a dressing. It's delicious, and you'll definitely find yourself buying larger containers of whole peppercorns to keep up.

The most effective way I've found to crack pepper is using a mortar and pestle. The pestle allows for maximum control for cracking corns, and it results in much less dust than, for example, using a spice grinder. And it's simple and easy to grind a tiny batch as needed.

For bigger jobs, I've on occasion used the time-honored method of crunching grains against a cutting board with the back of a small skillet or saucepan. It's time consuming, but it can result in some lovely, perfectly cracked grains while making little dust.

variation

SALTED LEMON PEPPER DRESSING

For an extra-punchy version of this dressing, you'll need a quarter of a Salted Lemon (page 64). Juice the pulp from the lemon and substitute it for some (or all, if you can muster up enough) of the lemon juice from the recipe. For the grated rind, simply mince the delicious salted lemon rind. You may want to decrease the amount of salt by half, then slowly add a pinch or two more to achieve the ideal amount of deliciousness.

CHIA NOTES

Superfood darlings, chia seeds are a common sight on grocery store shelves. The black chia seed is the most popular and will look similar to the cracked black pepper in this dressing. For a brighter dressing, use the less common (but nutritionally and taste-wise identical) white chia seed.

MORE VARIATIONS:

Leave out the added lemon zest and cracked peppers and instead try one of the following:

Herb Ranch: Add 3 tablespoons of mixed chopped fresh herbs: dill, basil, parsley, cilantro.

Avocado Lime: Pulse in ½ ripe avocado. Use lime juice instead of lemon.

Toasted Onion: Dry roast 2 tablespoons of dried onion bits in a small skillet over low heat. Stir frequently and watch carefully to avoid burning (burned onions will be bitter!). Add to the dressing along with the chia seeds.

Roasted Garlic: Replace fresh garlic clove with 3 to 4 roasted garlic cloves.

CUCUMBER DILL DRESSING

Makes 2 cups

TRY THIS IN:

Lazy Seitan Gyro Spinach Salad (page 204)

White Sweet Potato Salad with Spinach Zhug Dressing (page 198)

Zucchini and Chickpea Fattoush Salad (page 237)

Cucumbers / spring greens / asparagus / tomatoes / roasted potatoes

½ cup unroasted cashew pieces

½ cup cold water

1 tablespoon white wine vinegar

1 tablespoon lemon juice

2 garlic cloves, peeled

1 teaspoon kosher salt

¼ cup olive oil

½ cup grated, squeezed cucumber (no need to peel)

½ cup chopped fresh dill

1 scallion, minced

1 teaspoon whole black peppercorns, cracked

Inspired by Greek cucumber yogurt dish tzatziki, this cashew-based dressing is just thin enough to pour over greens, yet still thick enough to stand in as a dip for fresh veggies and pita.

Cucumbers are loaded with water, and you'll need to squeeze out as much liquid as possible to keep the dressing from becoming too watery. Many classic tzatziki recipes recommend gathering freshly grated cucumber into a few layers of paper towel to wring out the juices. Why not skip the paper towel and pack the cucumber into a small metal mesh colander set above a bowl, then use the back of a spoon to press out the juices? Bonus, you'll have a little shot of refreshing cucumber juice to power you through making the dressing.

Pour the cashew pieces into a small bowl and add enough hot tap water to cover with about 2 inches of water. Set aside to soak for 1 hour, or cover and soak overnight in the fridge.

Drain the cashews. Transfer to a blender and add the cold water, vinegar, lemon juice, garlic, and salt. Blend until the mixture is very smooth. Pulse in the oil, 1 tablespoon at a time, and pulse until the mixture is silky. Add the grated cucumber, dill, scallion, and pepper.

Pulse only a few times to break up the cucumber. Taste the mixture and season with more salt and lemon juice as needed.

For best results, chill the dressing for about 30 minutes prior to serving. Chock-full of herbs and so much fresh cucumber, a delicate dressing like this should be consumed within 12 hours of preparing for the best flavor.

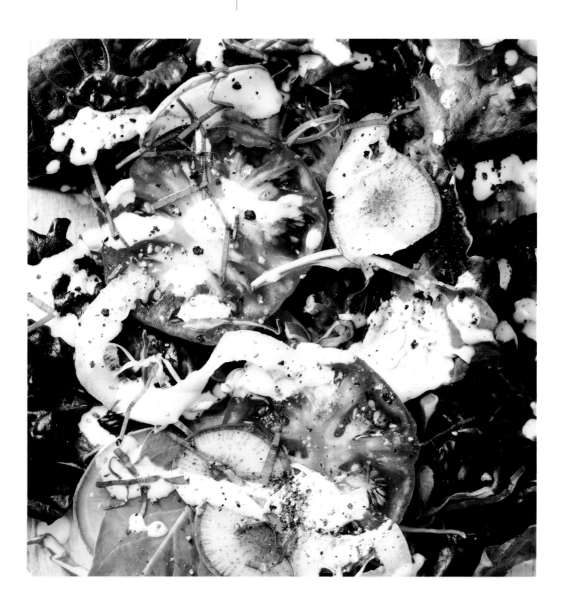

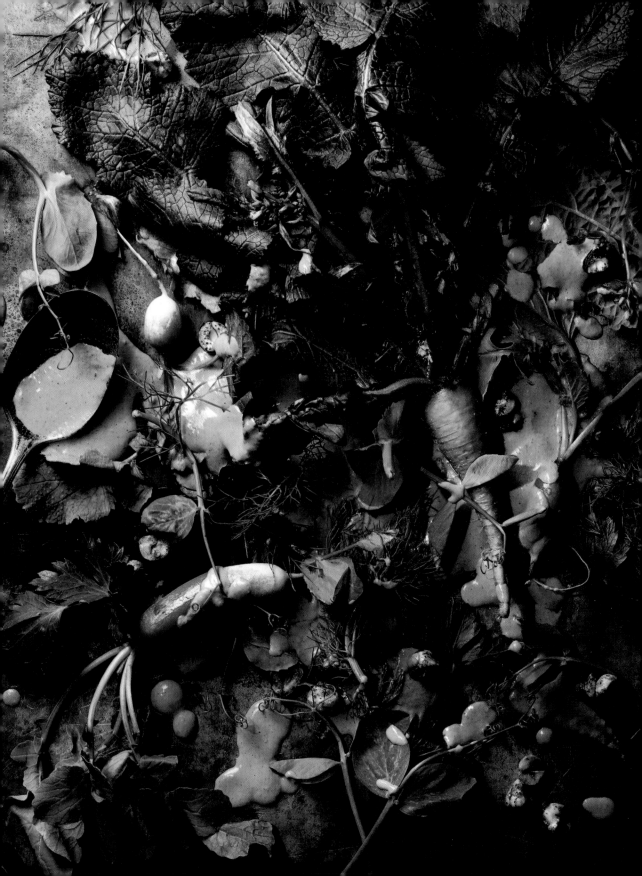

PEPITA GREENEST GODDESS DRESSING

Makes 1 cup

TRY THIS IN:

The Juicy Grilled Summer Days Peach Salad (page 155)

Buffalo Tofu, Butternut Squash, and Kale Bowl (page 176)

Spinach / corn / collards / zucchini / baby greens

⅓ cup pepitas, soaked for 30 minutes

½ cup unsweetened plain almond milk or favorite vegan plain unsweetened milk

2 tablespoons lemon juice

1 tablespoon sherry vinegar

½ teaspoon thyme or 1 teaspoon fresh thyme leaves

1 teaspoon kosher salt

½ cup spinach, watercress, or arugula, lightly packed

½ cup flat-leaf parsley, lightly packed

¼ cup fresh basil leaves, lightly packed

2 garlic cloves, peeled

2 teaspoons capers, drained

⅓ cup grape-seed oil or mild olive oil

Freshly ground black pepper to taste

You may be thinking, *Great. It will take 3 days for this boulder-hard avocado to ripen, so I have no avocados, so no green goddess dressing for me right now. Because every green goddess dressing requires avocados.* My friend, you are in luck. *This* creamy green dressing is packed with the herbal flavors of the California classic, but without mayonnaise, sour cream, or even avocado. Pepitas (shelled pumpkin seeds) add body instead of avocado, almond milk provides a creamy finish, and multiple acids perk up the fresh herbs. It's substantial enough to serve as a dip and can be loosened up with more almond milk for a pourable dressing.

Drain the pepitas and transfer to a blender with the almond milk, lemon juice, vinegar, thyme, and salt. Blend for 2 to 3 minutes until smooth, or at least as smooth as you can get the mixture. Add the spinach, parsley, basil, garlic, and capers. Blend until the dressing is bright green and silky.

Drizzle in the oil a little bit at a time, pulsing the mixture for 15 to 20 seconds at a time and scraping down the sides. Taste the mixture and season with black pepper or a dash more of kosher salt and lemon juice to adjust the seasoning. Pour into a small glass container. Cover and chill for an hour before serving. Whisk the dressing before serving and eat up within 2 days.

RED PEPPER AND ALMOND ROMESCO DRESSING

Makes 1½ cups

TRY THIS WITH:

Romaine lettuce / grilled leeks / roasted potatoes / roasted carrots

¼ cup blanched, sliced, or slivered almonds

1 cup diced roasted red pepper (about 2 roasted red peppers, homemade or from a jar, drained)

1 shallot, peeled and chopped

2 tablespoons red wine vinegar

1 tablespoon lemon juice

½ teaspoon sweet paprika

½ teaspoon dried oregano

¼ teaspoon dried thyme

1¼ teaspoons kosher salt

¼ cup olive oil

Thickened with puréed roasted red peppers and toasted almonds, this richly textured dressing is inspired by the timeless and totally vegan Romesco sauce. It's perfect on summery things like eggplant, tomatoes, and spicy greens.

Note that unlike most seed/nut-based dressings that need a serious blast of blending power to render them creamy, this veggie-based dressing requires a gentle hand with the blender. Pulse the red peppers only enough to make a chunky sauce; pulse too much (careful if using a Vitamix or Blendtec) and end up with a red pepper almond smoothie.

In a small skillet over medium heat, toast the almonds, stirring occasionally, for about 2 minutes, or until they smell fragrant and turn a light golden tan color.

Transfer the nuts to a food processor and pulse for about 10 seconds to break up the nuts, then add the roasted red pepper, shallot, vinegar, lemon juice, paprika, oregano, thyme, and salt. Pulse only a few times (don't over-blend!) into a chunky sauce, then stream in the oil and pulse to emulsify the sauce. Taste and adjust flavors with a dash or two more of salt and lemon juice, if desired. For the freshest flavor, use within 2 days, and keep chilled until ready to serve.

Tip ——————————

ROASTING A RED PEPPER
AT HOME

Roasting your own bell peppers is so easy, you'll never buy a jar again. Put whole, uncut peppers (about 2 per burner) directly on a gas burner and blast on high. Use long-handled tongs to occasionally rotate the pepper; cook until the skin is charred. Transfer to a mixing bowl, cover the top with a big dinner plate and leave undisturbed to steam for 5 minutes. When it is cool enough to touch, peel away the blackened skin (it will be messy!) and discard the seedy core. No gas range top? Roast the whole pepper on a cookie sheet in a 425°F oven until the skin is blistered and browned, then transfer to a mixing bowl as directed for stove-top peppers.

SULTRY PEANUT COCONUT DRESSING

Makes 1½ cups

TRY THIS WITH:

Peanut Avocado Brown Rice Crunch Bowl (page 211)

Spicy Cucumber and Curry Tofu Salad with Sticky Rice (page 212)

Steamed or roasted broccoli / steamed eggplant / blanched green beans / kale / spinach / thinly sliced green, red, or napa cabbage

½ cup full-fat Thai coconut milk, well stirred

⅓ cup warm water

2 tablespoons lime juice

2 tablespoons agave nectar or 2 dates, soaked and drained

½-inch piece ginger, peeled and minced

1 garlic clove, peeled and chopped

1 teaspoon sambal oelek paste

1 teaspoon tamari

1 teaspoon kosher salt

⅓ cup smooth, natural unsalted peanut butter

Impossible-to-resist, coconut milk–based peanut sauce feels right at home on hearty salads. While it may be pushing it a little to call this sauce a dressing, so many wonderful rice or noodle salads would not be the same without it. I've taken some liberties by opting for sweetness with either agave nectar or dates, the latter of which should be soaked in warm water for about 10 minutes before blending into the sauce.

When completely chilled, this dressing will thicken up thanks to the coconut milk and the peanut butter. Loosen it up a bit by whisking in a tablespoon or two of hot water before serving.

Blend together the coconut milk, warm water, lime juice, agave, ginger, garlic, sambal, tamari, and salt until smooth and emulsified. Scrape down the sides of the blender jar occasionally.

Add the peanut butter and pulse until smooth. Taste the dressing and add a teaspoon more of sambal, lime juice, or a pinch more of salt to sharpen up the flavors, if you like. Keep the dressing chilled until you're ready to use. Consume within 2 days.

DEEP DARK SESAME DRESSING

Makes about ¾ cup

DESIGNED FOR BUT NOT EXCLUSIVELY FOR:

General Tso's Tofu and Broccoli Salad (page 185)

Peking-Roasted Tofu Noodle Salad (page 217)

Thai Basil Spaghetti Squash with Curry Tofu (page 181)

Roasted Cabbage Steak with Peanut Sauce and Fried Shallots (page 186)

Soba noodles / cucumbers / butter lettuce / radishes / daikon

⅓ cup hoisin sauce

2 tablespoons rice vinegar

1½ teaspoons toasted sesame oil

1 garlic clove, minced

¼ teaspoon Chinese 5-spice powder

¼ teaspoon hot mustard powder

3 tablespoons grape-seed oil

Inspired by the rich, dark stir-fry sauces of lots of comforting Chinese take-out dishes, this sauce gets a sweet and umami-loaded boost from hoisin, the complex molasses-like sauce that gives so many Chinese stir-fry dishes their particular sweet-salty-savory richness, and it's my favorite on General Tso's Tofu and Broccoli Salad.

In a small mixing bowl or large measuring cup, whisk together everything except the oil. Then drizzle in the oil a little at a time, whisking until the mixture is smooth and emulsified. Use immediately!

WASABI MISO LIME DRESSING

Makes just over ⅓ cup

A GOOD ONE WITH:

Peanut Avocado Brown Rice Crunch Bowl (page 211)

Sriracha Tofu Lettuce Wraps with Peanut Dressing (page 169)

Thai Basil Spaghetti Squash with Curry Tofu (page 181)

Protein-Packed Salad for Breakfast (page 191)

2 tablespoons freshly squeezed lime juice

1 tablespoon rice vinegar

1 tablespoon agave nectar

2 teaspoons prepared wasabi paste

2 teaspoons white or yellow miso

Pinch white pepper, if using wasabi powder

¼ teaspoon kosher salt, or to taste

¼ cup mild olive oil or grape-seed oil

Cool and spicy with a fresh lime kick, this dressing was made for the Peanut Avocado Brown Rice Crunch Bowl but goes great with any Asian-inspired salad. This dressing uses an "intermediate" level of wasabi; use more or less depending on your preference. Make sure to use prepared wasabi paste (the ready-to-eat paste in a tube) instead of powdered wasabi for a lovely pastel-green dressing with a cool spicy kick.

In a small mixing bowl or large measuring cup, whisk together everything except the oil. Then drizzle in the oil a little at a time, whisking until the mixture is smooth and emulsified. Use promptly to prevent the dressing from separating.

GINGER GARLIC FIRE DRESSING

Makes ⅓ cup

TRY THIS WITH:

Orange Collard Greens, Corn, and Black-Eyed Peas (page 173)

The Bright and Spicy Spring Asparagus Salad (page 151)

Romaine lettuce / shaved red bell pepper / peanuts / black beans

2-inch piece fresh ginger, peeled

2 garlic cloves, peeled

½ teaspoon mustard powder or hot Chinese mustard powder

1 teaspoon kosher salt

2 tablespoons lime juice

1 tablespoon apple cider vinegar

1 tablespoon agave nectar (optional)

½ teaspoon toasted sesame oil

¼ cup mild olive oil or grape-seed oil

Inspired by the bright and gingery dressing on the collard salad at NuVegan Café in D.C., this bright and gingery sibling of Wasabi Miso Lime Dressing (page 56) is very, very gingery and garlicky, with a pucker-up one-two punch of lime juice and apple cider vinegar. The warm aroma of toasted sesame oil and mustard powder makes it a natural in Asian-inspired salads, but it's great for any salad loaded with crunchy fresh greens.

Blend together everything except the oil until smooth. Drizzle the oil into the blender jar and pulse until the mixture is smooth and emulsified. Use promptly to prevent the dressing from separating.

CARROT GINGER DRESSING

Makes ¾ cup

POUR IT ALL OVER:

Peanut Avocado Brown Rice Crunch Bowl (page 211)

Mustard Greens Tabbouleh with Almonds and Roasted Chickpeas (page 222)

The Bright and Spicy Spring Asparagus Salad (page 151)

½ cup finely grated, peeled carrot

½-inch piece ginger, peeled

2 tablespoons rice vinegar

1 tablespoon freshly squeezed lemon juice

1 tablespoon light agave nectar

1 tablespoon white miso

½ teaspoon kosher salt, or to taste

¼ cup avocado, sunflower, or grape-seed oil

1 teaspoon toasted sesame oil

1 tablespoon toasted white sesame seeds

Brilliantly orange and full of sweet carrot flavor, variations on carrot ginger miso dressings have been much sought after for years; my favorite version is a little different from the typical Japanese restaurant version and benefits from a good, thorough blending with a high-speed blender.

In a blender, pulse everything together except the oils and sesame seeds until smooth. Drizzle in the oils a little at a time, pulsing until the mixture is smooth and emulsified, then add the sesame seeds and pulse once. Taste dressing and season with additional rice vinegar, a dash of agave, or salt as needed. Keep chilled until ready to use; for the best flavor, use within a day of preparing.

ROASTED PICO DE GALLO DRESSING

Makes 1½ cups

MAKE THIS ONE FOR:

All-Day Breakfast Nacho Salad Bowl (page 192)

Orange Collard Greens, Corn, and Black-Eyed Peas (page 173)

Protein-Packed Salad for Breakfast (page 191)

Avocado / chickpeas / roasted zucchini / chopped scallions

1 pint cherry tomatoes, rinsed and dried

½ cup cilantro, chopped

½ cup diced white onion

1 fresh jalapeño, minced, or ¼ teaspoon chipotle powder

4 teaspoons lime juice

1 teaspoon agave nectar (optional)

1 teaspoon kosher salt

2 tablespoons extra-virgin olive oil

When a recipe absolutely requires fresh tomatoes, cherry tomatoes are my standby. Unlike larger "no flavor" standard supermarket tomatoes, or pricy hothouse tomatoes, these tiny round tomatoes typically pack a lot of flavor all year round.

Place a dry cast-iron skillet in the oven and preheat over high broil for 1 minute. Pull out the hot pan (don't forget your oven mitt), add the whole, dry cherry tomatoes, and return to the broiler. Broil for another 5 to 8 minutes to blister the tomatoes; the skins should look partially charred, and some (if not all) will have softened and split open and released some tomato juices. Turn off the broiler, remove the pan, and pour the tomatoes into a blender. Transfer the remaining ingredients except the oil to a blender and pulse until smooth. Stream in the oil. For the best flavor, use as soon as possible, within a day of preparing.

SUN-DRIED TOMATO DRESSING

Makes ⅓ cup

DAMNED GOOD ON:

Crunchy Eggplant Parm Salad (page 207)

Roasted Tomato Chickpea Pasta Salad with Caesar Walnuts (page 231)

Lazy Seitan Gyro Spinach Salad (page 204)

Fresh ripe summer tomatoes / cucumbers / marinated zucchini / robust crinkly spinach

4 sun-dried tomato halves, soaked

1 cup hot water

2 tablespoons sherry vinegar or balsamic vinegar

1 garlic clove, peeled

½ teaspoon dried oregano

½ teaspoon dried basil

Pinch red pepper flakes, or to taste

½ teaspoon kosher salt, or to taste

A few twists of black pepper

¼ cup mild olive oil or grape-seed oil

1 to 2 teaspoons agave nectar (optional)

Rich in big fat tomato flavor, blending sun-dried tomatoes into dressing is an easy way to add both body and abundant umami flavor to any salad. Sun-dried tomatoes are loaded with concentrated sweetness, but if your tomatoes taste a tad sharp, add a teaspoon of agave nectar to balance out the flavors. While the pico de gallo dressing is all about just-picked freshness, this dressing has the robust flavors of a marinara sauce simmered on the stove all day.

In a small bowl, cover the dried tomatoes with the hot water and soak for 10 minutes. When the tomatoes are softened, drain but reserve the soaking liquid. Remove the halves and roughly chop.

Blend together the soaked tomatoes, ½ cup of the reserved tomato soaking water, vinegar, garlic, dried herbs, red pepper flakes, salt, and pepper into a chunky sauce. Pulse in a tablespoon of oil at a time until emulsified. If you prefer a thinner dressing, drizzle in a tablespoon at a time of reserved tomato soaking water to achieve a consistency you're happy with. Taste and adjust seasoning with a pinch more salt and if too tart, add the agave nectar to taste. Use within 3 days.

HOLLYHOCK DRESSING

Makes ½ cup

1 fat garlic clove, peeled

½ teaspoon kosher salt

2 tablespoons apple cider vinegar

1 to 2 teaspoons maple syrup (optional)

1 tablespoon tamari

1 tablespoon lemon juice

¼ cup nutritional yeast flakes

A few twists of black pepper

¼ cup extra-virgin olive oil

This tawny, umami-loaded dressing has an ingredient list that reads like a hippie's shopping list from 1978. But I was first introduced to this dressing during a weeklong silent meditation retreat for punks in 2016 and since learned of its way-back origins at the famous Hollyhock retreat center on Cortes Island (never been, but if it's as good as the dressing, then I'm there). Make no mistake! It's held up over the decades for a reason and deserves wider appreciation beyond vegans and nooch (nutritional yeast's nickname) lovers, because it's freakin' delicious.

My take has a bit of lemon juice to complement the apple cider vinegar and scales down the proportions just a little. And if you're thinking this would be a great time to use that old-school bottle of Bragg Liquid Aminos in place of tamari? Then, my friend, you are a genius.

Blend together the garlic, salt, vinegar, maple syrup, tamari, lemon juice, 1 tablespoon of water, nutritional yeast, and black pepper. Blend until smooth and the yeast flakes have completely dissolved. Now drizzle in the oil a little at a time, pulsing until the mixture is smooth and emulsified.

If you prefer a thinner dressing, add 1 to 2 more tablespoons of water. Traditional recipes for this dressing add quite a bit of additional water, even as much as a cup, perhaps as a way to introduce eaters new to the zesty ways of nooch. But if you love nutritional yeast and know its pleasures, you'll probably agree this dressing is fine without being watered down. Use within 3 days for the best flavor.

NEW CATALINA DRESSING

Makes 1⅓ cup

MY FAVORITE WITH:

All-Day Breakfast Nacho Salad Bowl (page 192)

Blackened Tempeh Reuben Salad (page 179)

Sriracha Ranch Salad Party (page 165)

Red cabbage / cucumber / iceberg, butter, Boston lettuce / radishes / orange segments / sunflower seeds

1 cup canned diced tomatoes, with juices

2 tablespoons red wine vinegar

1 tablespoon agave nectar

1 shallot, peeled and chopped

2 teaspoons Dijon mustard

½ teaspoon smoked sweet paprika

¼ teaspoon cayenne pepper

1 teaspoon kosher salt

A few twists of freshly ground black pepper

3 tablespoons mild olive oil

Retro-cool Catalina and French dressings have fascinated me ever since I could shake a bottle of dressing. French relies on ketchup or tomato paste for a creamy orange hue (and in this book, tahini for lushness, page 42), and dark red Catalina dressing requires juicy tomatoes with a hint of spice. My version uses canned tomatoes (a fantastic emulsifier for dressings) for sweetness and convenience (also pretty sweet)! Want additional smoky richness? Use canned roasted tomatoes.

Blend everything together everything except the oil. Then drizzle in the oil a little at a time, pulsing until the mixture is smooth and emulsified. Use within a day of preparing.

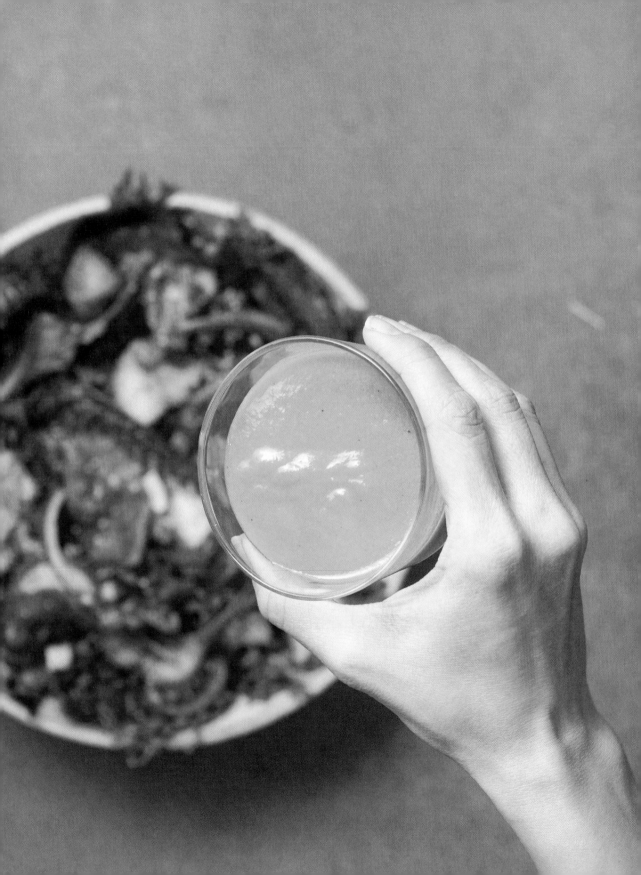

SALTED LEMONS

Makes 2 lemons, enough for 4 to 6 recipes

ESSENTIAL FOR:

Oil-Free Cashew Lemon Pepper Dressing (page 46)

Oregano Garlic Lemon Vinaigrette (page 69)

Zucchini and Chickpea Fattoush Salad (page 237)

Green Again Soup with Tahini Miso Slaw (page 253)

Anything, really, when a boost of fresh savory lemon flavor is needed

2 large, thick-skinned organic lemons

½ cup kosher salt

The complex flavors of preserved lemons add magic to so many recipes. Just a little bit of minced fermented lemon adds a uniquely sour, salty, and bitter hit to any dish, especially refreshing in salads.

The process of fermenting lemons with salt turns hard, bitter lemon rind tender. Like anything preserved and fermented, real-deal preserved lemons take weeks to ripen, but sometimes your salad needs the punch of a preserved lemon today. You're in luck here. This process is so easy and requires planning just the day before; you can keep one or two in the freezer for whenever a dish needs that kick of salty-sour sweetness.

The lemons are salted just like the traditional method, yet instead of packing them into brine and forgetting about them for weeks, these lemons are sealed in a zip-top bag and frozen overnight. Freezing breaks down the cell walls of the lemons, and the exchange of tenderizing salt can do its work in a fraction of the time.

These speed lemons don't have all the complexity that real fermented lemons do, but they add unmistakable zesty flavor and are so easy, why not give it a go?

Wash and pat dry the lemons. Starting on the stem end of the fruit, slice each lemon lengthwise ¾ of the way down. Keep ½ inch of this end unsliced; this will help keep the lemon whole and in one piece. Slice again at a 90-degree angle from the previous cut, stopping ½ inch from the bottom. You should have an *X* cut into deep into the one end of each of the lemons.

Stuff as much kosher salt as possible into the cuts, filling the insides of the lemon with a ridiculous amount of salt. Rub the outsides of the lemons with more salt. Pack the lemons into a zip-top bag, pouring in any remaining salt. Press out excess air and seal the top of the bag.

Freeze overnight, for at least 12 hours. When ready to use, remove a lemon and thaw in a small bowl for a minute or two on the kitchen counter. When it's softened up a little, tear off a section of the lemon. Freeze again any remaining lemon for later.

Typically, the fleshy rind of the preserved lemons is used. If you like, slice away the pulpy interior. I like to press any juice from this salty pulp and use immediately in a recipe.

To use the salted rind, mince the rind. Mince the lemon, measure, and then use. The average organic lemon with a fairly thick rind should yield a heaping tablespoon of minced rind per quarter section. Use the frozen lemons within 3 months for the best flavor.

variation

SHAVED SALTED LEMONS

Can't even wait overnight? Shave a lemon on a mandoline into wispy, papery-thin slices. Toss with a heaping teaspoon of kosher salt, rubbing the salt thoroughly into the slices. Set aside for 15 minutes to tenderize and use as you would overnight freezer lemons.

1-MINUTE VINAIGRETTES FOR EVERY DAY

OK, buying a bottle may be the simplest way to dressing. But this ain't far from it, on the easy train, and it's homemade—so infinitely better. Simple, and slightly beyond simple, vinaigrettes take only minutes. Use these dressings right away; you can always make more!

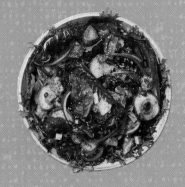

KEEP IT SIMPLE VINAIGRETTE

Makes about ½ cup

2 tablespoons balsamic vinegar, apple cider vinegar, red wine or white wine vinegar, or rice vinegar

1 tablespoon lemon juice or lime juice

2 teaspoons agave nectar

¾ teaspoon salt, or to taste

A few twists of freshly ground black pepper

¼ cup mild olive oil or grape-seed oil

The name says it all: This is the simplest way to season any bounty of greens. The kind of vinegar you choose shapes the flavors and provides so many options with the same recipe.

Red wine vinegar and balsamic vinegar have their own sweet, berry-like notes and are unmistakably Italian in flavor and character. White wine vinegar is more neutral, but the crisp white wine notes temper the acidity. Apple cider vinegar is rich, fruity, and slightly malty and has a chic health-food vibe that's forever in style.

A final tablespoon of citrus juice, while another acidic ingredient, adds layers of fruit, some sweetness, and a particular fruity sourness to the powerful single-note punch of vinegar.

In a small mixing bowl or large measuring cup, whisk together everything except the oil. Then drizzle in the oil a little at a time, whisking until the mixture is smooth and emulsified. Use promptly, as the dressing will naturally start to separate.

BRIGHT AND TANGY LEMON MAPLE VINAIGRETTE

Makes about ½ cup

2 tablespoons freshly squeezed lemon juice

1 tablespoon apple cider vinegar

1 tablespoon maple syrup

1 teaspoon minced shallot

½ teaspoon lemon zest

½ teaspoon mustard powder

½ teaspoon salt, or to taste

3 tablespoons mild olive oil

Lemon and apple cider vinegar are fruity and tangy partners in this classy dressing. Switch out the kind of mustard for an entirely different effect, as in the Maple Mustard Shallot Vinaigrette.

In a small mixing bowl or large measuring cup, whisk together everything except the oil. Then drizzle in the oil a little at a time, whisking until the mixture is smooth and emulsified. Use promptly to prevent the dressing from separating.

OREGANO GARLIC LEMON VINAIGRETTE

Makes about ½ cup

---

1 garlic clove

1 teaspoon kosher salt

2 tablespoons lemon juice

1 tablespoon red wine vinegar or white wine vinegar

1 teaspoon dried oregano or 1 tablespoon fresh oregano, minced

⅓ cup extra-virgin olive oil

Simple and zesty and ready to pour all over any Mediterranean or summertime-spirited salad, ideal for dressing piles of crisp greens or a small heap of ripe tomatoes.

In a mortar and pestle, mash together the garlic and salt into a paste. Scoop the paste into a small mixing bowl or large measuring cup. Pour in the remaining ingredients except the oil.

Drizzle in the oil a little at a time, whisking until the mixture is smooth and emulsified. Use promptly to prevent the dressing from separating.

variation

WHITE BALSAMIC DRESSING
Swap in white balsamic vinegar in place of the wine vinegars for a fruity, aromatic version of this dressing.

POMEGRANATE VINAIGRETTE
Substitute 1 tablespoon pomegranate molasses for the vinegar.

MAPLE MUSTARD SHALLOT VINAIGRETTE

Makes ⅓ cup

2 tablespoons Dijon mustard

1 tablespoon maple syrup

1 tablespoon white wine vinegar

1 large shallot, peeled and minced

¼ teaspoon dried thyme

½ teaspoon kosher salt, or to taste

A few twists of freshly ground black pepper

3 tablespoons mild olive oil

"One Vinaigrette to Rule Them All" would be the subtitle for this recipe, if recipes got subtitles. This is the skeleton key of salad dressing: The sweetness from maple and the full-bodied tang and richness from the mustard unlock the potential of so many salads. A favorite you'll find uses for time and time again.

In a small mixing bowl or large measuring cup, whisk together everything except the oil. Then drizzle in the oil a little at a time, whisking until the mixture is smooth and emulsified. Use promptly to prevent the dressing from separating.

BALSAMIC DIJON VINAIGRETTE

Makes about ⅓ cup

1 fat garlic clove, peeled

½ teaspoon kosher salt

1 tablespoon balsamic vinegar

1 tablespoon Dijon mustard

2 teaspoons agave nectar

A few twists of black pepper

¼ cup extra-virgin olive oil

Two reliable ingredients create yet another vinaigrette that sparks up any salad. Whisk it like crazy to ensure it's perfectly emulsified, and enjoy a smooth and rich dressing that eagerly clings onto greens and tomatoes.

Mash together the garlic with the salt in a mortar and pestle into a chunky paste. Scoop the paste into a small mixing bowl or large measuring cup, and add the remaining ingredients except the oil. Whisk it all together, then drizzle in the oil a little bit at a time, whisking until the mixture is smooth and emulsified.

This dressing is very stable and can be chilled overnight without separating, but for the best flavor, it should be used within a day of preparing.

THE BEST ORANGE
BALSAMIC VINAIGRETTE

Makes ½ cup

¼ cup freshly squeezed orange juice

½ teaspoon orange zest

1 tablespoon balsamic vinegar or white balsamic vinegar

1 teaspoon agave nectar

1 teaspoon Dijon mustard

1 teaspoon minced shallot or minced garlic

½ teaspoon kosher salt

A few twists of freshly ground black pepper

¼ cup extra-virgin olive oil

The Balsamic Dijon Vinaigrette is like a weekday little black dress for salads, but this version is the shorter black dress with a plunging neckline, adding major sex appeal to all manner of salad from fluffy greens to pasta and roasted vegetables. Fresh citrus flavor and a touch of shallot add sparkle to the mighty flavor pairing of Dijon and balsamic vinegar.

In a small mixing bowl or large measuring cup, whisk together everything except the oil. Then drizzle in the oil a little at a time, whisking until the mixture is smooth and emulsified. Taste and season with a little more salt or vinegar if needed. Use promptly to prevent the dressing from separating, and consume within a day of making for the best flavor.

SAVORY PLANT-BASED PROTEIN TOPPINGS

What goes on top of the leafy greens and other substantial elements can make or break your home salad bar. Naked diced celery, cold watery cubes of plain tofu, raw sunflower seeds, sliced beets poured straight out of the can . . . these are the business of an ordinary lackluster salad bar. The toppers here, however, are the flavor-rich, umami-loaded, roasted and toasted, memorable islands of pleasure that drift above the fresh veggies, grains, and greens (sorry, canned beets and naked celery).

Don't fret—you'll get your classics: croutons (and I *love* bread) and many toasted candied nuts. But vegan salads offer a unique opportunity: to create the salty, fatty, plant-based replacements for cheese, bacon, or other standard things you'll find on a salad, along with some unexpected items—cornbread croutons, walnuts that taste like Caesar salad, pickled red onions, fried shallots, or cheesy golden almonds.

Just one or two of these toppings make the entire salad leap to life. Make a few and stock your kitchen for a week of incredible salad adventures.

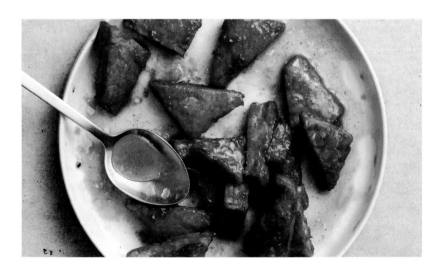

MIGHTY AND FLAVORFUL
TOFU, TEMPEH, AND SEITAN

Robust, chewy, full of flavor, no matter what your base, this is the protein-packed center of attention every full-meal salad deserves. Tofu and its fermented kin in the traditional soy foods family, tempeh, are easy to season with juicy marinades and take up flavor beautifully. Seitan, the lesser known of the three, is a traditional meat-like food (made long before the advent of the huge selection of fake meats) made from wheat gluten; if you can eat gluten, seitan is your salad's best friend.

There are dozens of ways to season tofu, tempeh, and seitan. Marinades must be packed with flavor; plenty of garlic, helpful acids such as citrus juice or vinegar, and a healthy dash of salt or soy sauce (not the time to be subtle). The following marinades will help you make plant-based, protein-rich main-attraction salads from humble supermarket ingredients. The method is the same for all flavors and marinade recipes. Once cooked, serve tofu cubes slightly cooled, room temp, or chilled on a salad. Double, triple, quadruple the recipes for a massive batch of ready-to-eat, fully flavored tofu to last throughout the week.

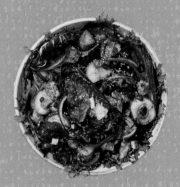

MARINATED BAKED TOFU

Makes 2 entrée salad servings of flavorful tofu (about 3 cups diced)

1 (15- to 16-ounce) block firm or extra-firm tofu

1 recipe marinade

Why bake tofu? I love baking tofu, as it's mostly hands-off (just slide into the oven, flip only once), and the tofu pieces are evenly firm and chewy. It does take longer than stove-top tofu and heats up the kitchen, but it's a must if you are making large batches of tofu for the week.

Drain and press the tofu, either pressing the entire block in a tofu press or as directed (see Press That Tofu, page 76). If the entire block is pressed first, slice the pressed tofu into 12 slices.

Preheat the oven to 400°F. In an 11 x 7 x 2-inch baking dish, whisk all the ingredients for any marinades directly into the dish. No need to dirty an extra mixing bowl! If making the sliced baked tofu, arrange the slices in the dish (it's okay to overlap slices). Marinate the tofu slices for 5 minutes, flip them over once, and marinate for another 5 minutes.

If preparing the roasted tofu cubes, dice the sliced tofu into ½-inch cubes. Stir the cubes into the marinade and set aside to marinate for 20 minutes, stirring occasionally.

Bake sliced tofu for 30 to 35 minutes, flipping each sliced over once at about 20 minutes. The sliced tofu is done when the marinade has been absorbed and the cutlets are rich golden brown and sizzling. Roast diced tofu for about 30 minutes, stirring occasionally until the cubes are golden brown and firm.

FRIED OR GRILLED TOFU

More tender than chewy, fried marinated tofu is perfect when you need a small batch of tofu, fast. The tofu is rendered tender, and if grilled, it perhaps has some pretty grill marks too.

Preheat a cast-iron pan over medium heat until a drop of water sizzles on the surface. Spray or brush with your choice of high-heat cooking spray (peanut, high-heat canola, grape-seed oil). Place the tofu in a single layer, leaving a little room between pieces; if necessary, divide the tofu into two batches for even cooking. Fry for 3 to 4 minutes until golden brown on the edge, flip, and fry another 2 to 3 minutes to brown the other side. Pour a little marinade over the tofu and flip a few times until browned as you please. Repeat with any remaining tofu, drizzling with any remaining marinade after flipping once.

TOFU CARE AND FEEDING: TIPS

PRESS THAT TOFU

Pressing the water out of tofu helps transform it from flabby to fabulous. Once pressed, tofu drinks up marinades like a thirsty champ. The following method uses two cutting boards and clean kitchen towels, but small baking sheets and a bunch of paper towels works fine as well.

This method is cheap and uses what you already have, a double win. But if you love tofu and prepare it more than twice a week, get a tofu press. No more wasted paper towels or soggy wet dish towels! There are a few great tofu presses on the market. I prefer the design that sets the tofu into its own container (catching all the water), but models that rest in your sink to catch the drainage are well made and work great too.

Slice a block of firm or extra-firm tofu crosswise into 12 equal slices.

Cover a cutting bowl with a clean kitchen towel and arrange the slices on top. Do not overlap. Cover with another towel and top with another cutting board.

Prop your cutting board–tofu sandwich on an angle next to the edge of the sink. Add a few thick cookbooks or other heavy things on top of the cutting board and let it press for about 20 to 25 minutes. The excess water will drain into the nearby sink and press into the towels.

FREEZE THAT TOFU

Frozen tofu is a miracle! Once frozen tofu is completely thawed and drained, the tiny pockets of water that riddle tofu are set free, creating tofu with a uniquely chewy texture. This extra-absorbent tofu wicks up marinade all the way through each slice, for tofu loaded with flavor with each bite. Why don't we freeze tofu all the time, you may ask? We can! It just requires some planning, as a typical container of tofu needs at least 10 to 12 hours to completely freeze solid, then about 45 minutes to thaw. Get in the habit of having a few packages of tofu in your freezer and you'll be the master of super-tasty tofu, anytime.

To thaw tofu: Place a frozen container of tofu in a mixing bowl and put in the sink. Run cool water over the tofu, flipping occasionally, until thawed. Once removed from the package, give it a gentle squeeze to release more of the water, or press for about 20 minutes. Then use as the recipe directs.

MARINATED OR BAKED TEMPEH

Makes 2 servings

8-ounce package of tempeh

1 recipe marinade

Tempeh, the fermented soybean cake with a firm, hearty texture, works great with these marinades. Slice an 8-ounce package of tempeh into either strips or small triangles (slicing the cake in half first) about ½ inch thick.

Along with the marinade ingredients, whisk in the 2 tablespoons of water. The extra water provides the moisture to steam the tempeh as it cooks, helping it tenderize and absorb more of the marinade's flavor.

Heat a 10- to 12-inch cast-iron pan over medium heat, slick the bottom with high-heat cooking oil, such as refined canola or safflower, and make a single layer (don't overlap slices) of marinated tempeh strips on the bottom. Divide the tempeh into two batches to prevent crowding the pan, if necessary. Fry for 2 to 3 minutes, or just long enough to brown that side, flip over, and fry the other side just until browned (probably just 1 minute or a bit more). Drizzle with a little marinade and fry for 1 more minute until the tempeh has absorbed most of the marinade but looks still a little juicy.

MARINATED
PAN-FRIED SEITAN

Makes 2 servings

8 ounces seitan, store-bought or homemade (page 81)

1 recipe marinade

Any of these marinades can also be used with seitan, the meatiest of simple meat substitutes. These chunks of flavorful wheat gluten hold up to panfrying exceptionally well. Chewy strips of seitan are a favorite of mine in leafy salads too. The method for using seitan with these marinades is to slice the seitan (homemade or purchased) into ¼-inch-thick strips or pieces. Keep those pieces the same thickness to help it soak up marinades swiftly and for even cooking for each piece.

You'll want to panfry the marinated seitan rather than bake. Baking marinated cutlets can dry out these thin slices, and pan-fried seitan remains the juiciest.

Heat a cast-iron pan over medium heat, slick the bottom with high-heat cooking oil such as refined canola or safflower, and place a single layer of marinated seitan strips on the bottom. Fry for 2 to 3 minutes, or just long enough to brown that side, flip over, and fry the other side just until browned (probably just 1 minute or a bit more).

MARINATED ROASTED YUBA

Makes 2 servings

5-ounce package yuba (fresh) or
4 ounces yuba sticks (dried)

1 recipe marinade

Cooking spray

Yuba is a much-loved and appreciated soy food throughout Asia, but it's still just catching on in North America. It's essentially soy milk skin, a dense and chewy layer that forms on the surface of cooking soy milk (during the tofu-making process), that's lifted up and off the milk—think a big flat tofu-like noodle. Yuba dishes can be prepared from fresh yuba, or the yuba can be dried into thin strips to be rehydrated later.

If using dried yuba sticks, completely cover with water and soak overnight or for 8 hours until soft and pliable. When ready to marinate, firmly squeeze the sticks to release as much water as possible.

No need to soak fresh yuba—just remove it from the package! Then unfold the fresh yuba sheet once or twice, just to loosen up the layers; no need to completely unfold the sheet. Slice the yuba into strips about ¾ inch wide. Gently pull apart the strands and fluff them up a little.

Whisk together your choice of marinade ingredients in a large mixing bowl. Add the yuba strips and gently knead the strips into the marinade. Cover and marinate the strips for about 10 minutes.

Preheat the oven to 400°F. Line a large cookie sheet with parchment paper, and give the paper a little blast of cooking oil (preferably olive oil) spray. Arrange the strips in a single layer on the cookie sheet. Bake for 4 to 6 minutes, then flip each strip, and bake until the edges are very crisp and golden brown, another 4 minutes or so. Serve crisp and hot or chilled, and store in a tightly covered container in the fridge.

MARINATED
PAN-FRIED ABURAAGE

Makes 2 servings

4 to 6 ounces of aburaage

1 recipe marinade

Also spelled *aburage,* these thin pouches of fried tofu with pita-like pockets are essential in Japanese cuisine. They are ready to eat out of the package and require only a rinse with hot water to remove some of the excess oil. Used commonly for inari sushi and udon noodle dishes, they're also a good stand-in cut into thin strips for chewy, noodle-like tofu into salads. In a pinch, just pat dry rinsed aburaage and slice into thin noodles. Fried to a golden hue and chewy texture, they can jump headfirst into great leafy or rice-based salads.

While ready to eat, it's fun to marinate sliced aburaage to add a little extra flavor.

Whisk the marinade ingredients in a shallow bowl. Slice the aburaage into ½-inch-wide strips and fold into the marinade. Heat a 10- to 12-inch cast-iron pan over medium heat, slick the bottom with high-heat cooking oil, such as refined canola or safflower, and make a single layer (don't overlap slices) of aburaage strips on the bottom. Divide the aburaage into two batches to prevent crowding the pan, if necessary. Fry for 2 to 3 minutes, or just long enough to brown that side, flip over, and fry the other side just until browned (probably just 1 minute or a bit more). Drizzle with a little marinade.

Serve crisp and hot or chilled, and store in a tightly covered container in the fridge and eat up within 2 days.

READY-TO-EAT FLAVORED TOFU

Did you eat your last bite of tofu and forget to stock up? In a salad quandary? You may be fortunate to have baked, pressed, and flavored tofu in your supermarket refrigerated case. Hodo Soy (a wonderful Bay Area tofu company) makes a ready-to-use braised tofu brick, and several other brands feature ready-to-eat tofu in flavors such as sriracha, Jamaican jerk, or teriyaki that work great in salads. They are the perfect convenience food! I still make plenty of baked tofu at home, though, flavoring it as I please. Once you get the hang of it, it's just as convenient (and sometimes cheaper) than buying off-the-shelf flavored tofu.

STEAMED SEITAN CUTLETS

Makes 4 large cutlets, enough for 8 servings

1¾ cups (1 [10-ounce] package) vital wheat gluten flour

⅓ cup nutritional yeast

¼ cup chickpea flour

1 teaspoon ground sweet paprika

1¾ cups room-temperature, good-tasting vegetable broth

2 garlic cloves, minced or grated

3 tablespoons tamari

2 tablespoons extra-virgin olive oil

Easier than baking cookies from scratch, these simple, mildly seasoned seitan cutlets are steamed in 30 minutes and ready to hit the marinade once they are cool enough to slice. A refinement of the recipe for steamed seitan I've been perfecting for years, these chewy patties are a great beginner-friendly introduction to homemade seitan. If you can eat gluten, then seitan is a hearty way to embellish those salads with a truly homemade "almost like meat" vegan protein!

Tear or cut four 10-inch-wide pieces of aluminum foil. Set a steamer basket into a large 3-quart stockpot and add water, but only enough to leave about ½ inch under the basket. No water should touch the basket. Set the pot over medium-high heat and make the seitan dough while the water comes to a boil.

In a large bowl, stir together the vital wheat gluten flour, nutritional yeast, chickpea flour, and paprika. Form a well in the center. In a 1-quart glass measuring cup or smaller bowl, whisk together the vegetable broth, garlic, tamari, and olive oil.

Pour the liquid ingredients into the well of the dry ingredients. Stir vigorously with a rubber spatula; when all the broth has been absorbed and the dough pulls away from the sides of the bowl, use your hand to knead the dough for about 1 minute, or until all the ingredients are well mixed and the bowl looks mostly clean. Drop the dough onto a cutting board (no need to dust with flour) and knead for another minute. For the best texture results, knead the dough in one direction, using a folding and pressing motion with your palm.

Continued

Slice the dough into four equal pieces. Flatten and shape each piece into a rough oval about 1 inch thick. Place each piece in the center of a foil section. Seal each packet for steaming and bring the long edges of the foil together, fold once with a seam about ¼ inch wide, fold once again, and press together to secure the seam; there should still be a little room (about 1½ inches) from the foil tent and the seitan dough inside. Flatten and tightly crimp the short unfolded ends. Hopefully you now have a loose foil pouch of seitan with tightly sealed seams. Repeat three more times! Seitan expands as it steams, so a little room in the steaming pouch is essential.

Once the water is boiling in your steamer, arrange the foil pouches in a single layer (some overlap is okay) inside the basket. If they don't all fit, steam in two batches. Steam for about 30 minutes. To test doneness, use long-handled tongs to lift a seitan loaf out of the steamer, carefully unwrap the top (let the steam escape for a few seconds), and press the center; it should feel firm to the touch, not sticky like raw dough. When the seitan is done, remove and let cool inside their pouches until cool enough to slice. Store unused seitan in their pouches in a tightly covered container and chilled, and use within 1 week. Or freeze for 2 months!

THE MARINADES

Tofu, tempeh, and seitan are blank canvases and easy homemade marinades add that essential splash of flavor. Consider them dressings for vegan proteins before they're cooked!

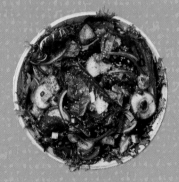

HOT SAUCE BUFFALO

Makes just over ½ cup

⅓ cup Frank's RedHot sauce (original) or similar vinegar-based hot sauce

3 tablespoons vegan butter or refined coconut oil, melted (see tip)

Our love affair with this pub-grub favorite can't be stopped (nor should it be). This is as simple as it gets, drenching vegan proteins in tangy vinegar-based hot sauce and a bit of vegan butter (or coconut oil). Grab hold of your celery sticks!

Whisk together the ingredients in an 11 x 7 x 2-inch, or similar-sized, baking dish. Add the prepared vegan protein and marinate for 10 minutes, flipping occasionally. Roast or panfry as directed for Mighty and Flavorful Tofu, Tempeh, and Seitan (page 74).

tip

The no-fuss way to melt the butter or coconut oil: Drop it into the baking dish and slide the dish into the oven as it preheats. In about 3 to 5 minutes, the solid fats will have melted, or will be melty enough, to whisk easily with the hot sauce.

SAVORY SESAME TAMARI

Makes ½ cup marinade

¼ cup tamari

2 tablespoons agave nectar

2 tablespoons mild-flavored oil (canola, grape-seed, or mild olive oil)

2 tablespoons sesame seeds

2 teaspoons toasted sesame oil

1 garlic clove, grated or smashed

Golden-brown tofu, seasoned with the irresistible and flexible flavors of tamari, sesame, and garlic. The obvious marinade for proteins for Asian salads, but tasty with a wide range of creamy and tomato-based dressings too.

Preheat the oven to 400°F. Whisk together all the ingredients in an 11 x 7 x 2-inch, or similar-sized, baking dish. Add the prepared vegan protein and marinate for 10 minutes, flipping occasionally. Roast as directed for Mighty and Flavorful Tofu, Tempeh, and Seitan (page 74).

KOREAN BBQ

Makes ⅔ cup

¼ cup good-quality soy sauce

2 tablespoons mild-flavored oil (canola, grapeseed, or mild olive oil)

2 tablespoons rice vinegar

1 tablespoon organic brown sugar

1 teaspoon toasted sesame oil

1 heaping teaspoon grated fresh ginger

2 garlic cloves, minced

½ teaspoon Korean red pepper powder or 1 small fresh red chile, minced

2 tablespoons sesame seeds

2 scallions, green part only, sliced paper thin

The queen of all soy sauce–based marinades, this Korean-style BBQ marinade checks all the boxes with bold soy-ginger-garlic-sesame flavors. Enhanced with acid and sugar, this marinade is ideal for tofu and seitan, but also excellent with tempeh and large, meaty shiitake mushroom caps.

Traditional Korean BBQ marinade also contains a little bit of shredded or juiced Asian pear (or other juicy, sweet-sour fruit), as the fruit sugar helps tenderize tough cuts of meat. As this marinade is designed for tender plant-based foods, I leave it out, but if you want that authentic touch, stir in ¼ cup finely shredded Asian pear.

Whisk together all the ingredients in an 11 x 7 x 2-inch, or similar-sized, baking dish. Add the prepared vegan protein and marinate for 10 minutes, flipping occasionally. Roast as directed for Mighty and Flavorful Tofu, Tempeh, and Seitan (page 74).

variation

KOREAN BBQ SHIITAKES

Cut the stems (reserve for homemade mushroom broth) from 1 pound of shiitake caps and marinate the caps for 1 hour, flipping occasionally. Roast or grill as directed for the tofu, stirring occasionally until juicy in the centers and slightly crisped on the edges.

PERUVIAN CHILE LIME

Makes ⅔ cup

¼ cup freshly squeezed lime juice

2 tablespoons tamari

2 tablespoons olive oil

2 teaspoons minced garlic

2 tablespoons aji amarillo paste

1 tablespoon agave nectar

½ teaspoon mustard powder

½ teaspoon ground cumin

½ teaspoon kosher salt

Peruvian aji amarillo (yellow chile) sauce is essential for capturing the Peruvian vibe of this subtly spicy and aromatic golden tofu (or tempeh or seitan). Look for jars of aji amarillo sauce wherever Latino or South American groceries are sold.

Whisk together all the ingredients in an 11 x 7 x 2-inch, or similar-sized, baking dish. Add the prepared vegan protein and marinate for 10 minutes, flipping occasionally. Roast or fry as directed for Mighty and Flavorful Tofu, Tempeh, and Seitan (page 74).

variation

ANCHO OR CHIPOTLE CHILE

Replace the aji amarillo sauce with 1 teaspoon ancho chile powder or chipotle chile powder for tofu or tempeh with *sabór Mexicano!*

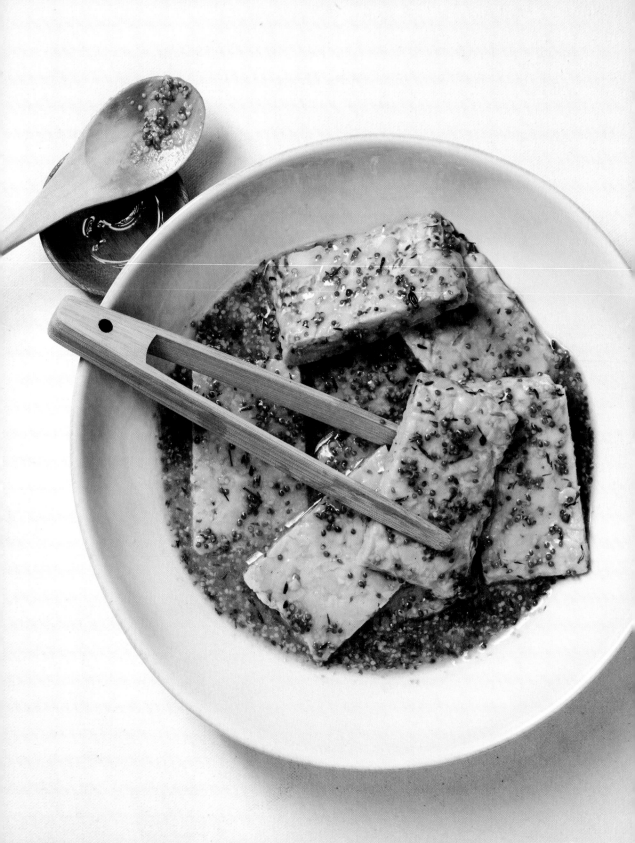

LEMON DIJON

Makes ¾ cup

¼ cup freshly squeezed lemon juice

¼ cup Dijon mustard

3 tablespoons olive oil

2 tablespoons agave nectar

1 teaspoon dried thyme or dried tarragon

Dijon mustard easily complements so many different dishes. Use this marinade for tofu or tempeh for French-inspired salads or any bright and crunchy leafy salad.

Whisk together all the ingredients in an 11 x 7 x 2-inch, or similar-sized, baking dish. Add the prepared vegan protein and marinate for 10 minutes, flipping occasionally. Roast or fry as directed for Mighty and Flavorful Tofu, Tempeh, and Seitan (page 74).

variation

OTHER MUSTARDS

In a pinch, stone-ground mustard or whole-grain mustard work great here too! A little less of a French vibe, but just as delicious.

SRIRACHA ORANGE

Makes ¾ cup

¼ cup sriracha sauce

2 tablespoons tamari

1 tablespoon agave nectar

1 garlic clove, minced

½ cup freshly squeezed orange juice

1 tablespoon mild-flavored oil (canola, grape-seed, or mild olive oil)

Arguably hotter than the Hot Sauce Buffalo (page 84), yet with irresistible fruity citrus sweetness and garlic sass that makes this a versatile way to flavor soy foods. Tempeh is my favorite protein for this marinade, but it's great for tofu and even seitan too.

Whisk together all the ingredients in an 11 x 7 x 2-inch, or similar-sized, baking dish. Add the prepared vegan protein and marinate for 10 minutes, flipping occasionally. Roast or panfry as directed for Mighty and Flavorful Tofu, Tempeh, and Seitan (page 74).

SWEET LIME CURRY

Makes ⅔ cup

¼ cup freshly squeezed lime juice (or bottled is okay; see note on page 28)

2 tablespoons coconut sugar or dark agave nectar

2 tablespoons melted coconut oil

1 tablespoon tamari

1 teaspoon mild curry powder

½ teaspoon kosher salt

The mellow curry flavor of this marinade, balanced with coconut sugar and lime, transforms vegan proteins into the superstar of any Thai, Vietnamese, or Southeast Asian salad; it's also fantastic in bahn mi sandwiches.

Whisk together all the ingredients in an 11 x 7 x 2-inch, or similar-sized, baking dish. Add the prepared vegan protein and marinate for 10 minutes, flipping occasionally. Roast or grill as directed for Mighty and Flavorful Tofu, Tempeh, and Seitan (page 74).

TAHINI MISO

Makes about ¾ cup

1/3 cup tahini

2 tablespoons white miso

3 tablespoons lemon juice

2 tablespoons olive oil

2 tablespoons water

1 teaspoon grated fresh ginger

1 garlic clove, pressed or grated

Unlike the other marinades, this silky tahini sauce bakes into a scrumptious fatty crust around the roasted protein that *is* irresistible! Great with Middle Eastern salads.

Whisk together all the ingredients in an 11 x 7 x 2-inch, or similar-sized, baking dish. Add the prepared vegan protein and marinate for 10 minutes, flipping occasionally. Roast as directed for Mighty and Flavorful Tofu, Tempeh, and Seitan (page 74).

variation

ZA'ATAR TOFU

Omit ginger. Add to the marinade 1 tablespoon za'atar seasoning. Sprinkle the cutlets with an additional dusting of za'atar before roasting.

GOLDEN CORIANDER BIRD

Makes 1 cup

½ cup vegetable broth, white wine, or lager beer

2 tablespoons olive oil

2 tablespoons nutritional yeast

1 tablespoon organic brown sugar

1 tablespoon soy sauce

1 tablespoon apple cider vinegar

1 teaspoon garlic powder

½ teaspoon sweet paprika

½ teaspoon kosher salt

¼ teaspoon ground pepper

¼ teaspoon ground turmeric

¼ teaspoon ground cumin

¼ teaspoon ground coriander

A sweet and aromatic marinade for roasted vegan protein that blends seamlessly into many cuisines, perhaps a little bit like a homemade faux roasted chicken breast. This plentiful marinade is especially handy for flavoring tofu that's been frozen and thawed; the spongy thawed texture drinks up the marinade unlike anything else. If you want to use tempeh or seitan, it's right at home there too. No matter your protein, it fits right into salads, sandwiches, or thinly sliced as a garnish on soups.

Whisk together all the ingredients in an 11 x 7 x 2-inch, or similar-sized, baking dish. Add the prepared vegan protein and marinate for 10 minutes, flipping occasionally. Roast or panfry as directed for Mighty and Flavorful Tofu, Tempeh, and Seitan (page 74).

MAPLE ALMOST LIKE BACON

Makes just under ½ cup

3 tablespoons mild olive oil or melted coconut oil

2 tablespoons tamari

2 tablespoons maple syrup

1 teaspoon smoked paprika

½ teaspoon chipotle powder

1 teaspoon kosher salt

There are many ways to bacon up vegan proteins and vegetables, and I've tried many. And I love them all! This marinade skips the ever-popular liquid smoke in favor of a little smoked paprika and a dash of chipotle powder. Good with any vegan protein, this marinade is especially good with yuba (see page 79) and frozen, thawed tofu (for that chewy and substantial texture). But whatever your protein choice, this spicier-than-bacon fix adds a kick to just about anything.

Whisk together all the ingredients in an 11 x 7 x 2-inch, or similar-sized, baking dish. Add the prepared vegan protein and marinate for 10 minutes, flipping occasionally. Roast or panfry as directed for Mighty and Flavorful Tofu, Tempeh, and Seitan (page 74).

OVEN-FRIED
BREAKFAST TOFU BITES

Makes 3 cups, about 2 to 3 generous servings

1 (15- to 16-ounce) block extra-firm tofu, pressed for 20 minutes and drained (see page 76 for tips on pressing tofu)

2 tablespoons lemon juice

2 tablespoons olive oil

1 tablespoon white miso

1 teaspoon mustard powder

¼ teaspoon ground turmeric

¼ teaspoon paprika

¼ teaspoon garlic powder

¼ teaspoon black salt (kala namak)

3 tablespoons nutritional yeast

Freshly ground pepper

Kosher salt or a few twists from a salt grinder

These chewy roasted cubes of golden, nutritional-yeasty tofu have a hint of Indian black salt (kala namak) for that egg-like taste: Some people love it, but if that's not you, leave it out. This "roasted tofu scramble" is just sturdy and assertive enough for breakfast salads and other brunch foods, and it is right at home in a pile of leafy greens. These bites were created with the All-Day Breakfast Nacho Salad Bowl (page 192) in mind, but are just as great rolled up in a tortilla for breakfast burritos.

Dice the pressed tofu into ½-inch cubes. In a mixing bowl, stir together the marinade ingredients into a creamy paste. Add the diced tofu and use a rubber spatula to gently stir to coat every piece with the marinade, but take care not to mash up the cubes. Cover the tofu and refrigerate for 1 hour or overnight.

Preheat the oven to 400°F. Line a large cookie sheet with parchment paper or foil.

Spread the tofu in a single layer, leaving a little space between the cubes to encourage browning. Bake for 20 to 25 minutes, flipping the cubes halfway. The tofu is ready when the edges are browned and crusty. Serve hot, warm, or cold.

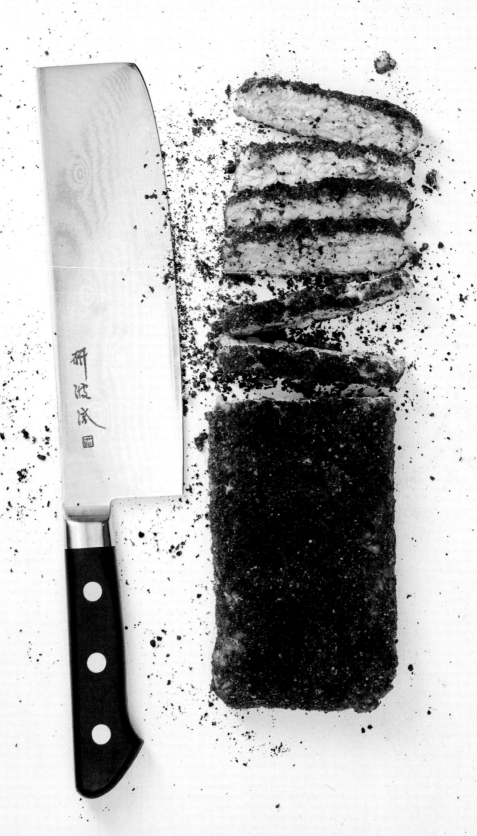

WHOLE-LOAF BLACKENED TEMPEH PASTRAMI

Makes 1 whole loaf, ideal for slicing thinly

PASTRAMI RUB

2 tablespoons black peppercorns

2 tablespoons coriander seeds

1 tablespoon yellow mustard seeds

1 tablespoon fennel seeds

1 tablespoon smoked paprika

1 tablespoon minced dried onion

1 tablespoon minced dried garlic

1 tablespoon kosher salt

TEMPEH

2 tablespoons brown sugar

1 tablespoon kosher salt

8 ounce package tempeh

At last, a whole block of juicy tempeh, slathered in pastrami spices and blackened in a cast-iron pan just like fancy BBQ chefs do. This hearty and spice-loaded tempeh creation is so rewarding to make, look at, and slice thinly to drape over leafy greens. My recipe testers opted to make double batches of the spice mix and tempeh and recommend you do the same! Don't skip out on the brown sugar "bath," as this is essential for plumping up the tempeh and preparing it to bond with the semi-authentic pastrami spice blend. Naturally, this is perfect with Horseradish Hemp Dressing (page 34) on a bed of thinly sliced red cabbage and whole-grain croutons.

In a spice grinder (or pound in a mortar and pestle), pulse together the black pepper, coriander, mustard seeds, and fennel seeds just to coarsely ground. Don't pulverize to a powder; you'll still want a gritty texture to the mix. Transfer to a small container and stir in the paprika, dried onion, dried garlic, and salt. Spread half of the spice mixture on a dinner plate.

In a 10-inch stainless steel skillet, combine the brown sugar and kosher salt with 2 cups of water. Bring to a rapid simmer over medium heat, add the tempeh, and simmer for 5 minutes. Flip the tempeh over and simmer another 5 minutes and turn off the heat.

Use a wide spatula to gently lift the tempeh (careful, that's hot, wet tempeh!) from the simmering water and place it onto the bed of spices, and layer the other half of the spices over the tempeh. Pat the spices into the surface

Continued

of the tempeh. Flip over and continue to pat the tempeh with a thorough coating of spices. Heat a cast-iron pan over medium-high heat.

Wipe a thin layer of high-heat cooking oil (such as canola or high-heat safflower) over the pan and add the tempeh. Cook without flipping over for at least 5 minutes, or until this side is charred. Flip over and repeat on the other side. It will get smoky in the kitchen, so crank the fan or open a window!

Use the large spatula to carefully lift the tempeh off the pan and transfer to a plate. Slice thinly and enjoy right away, or chill and slice for salads. It is best if it's eaten within 2 days of preparing.

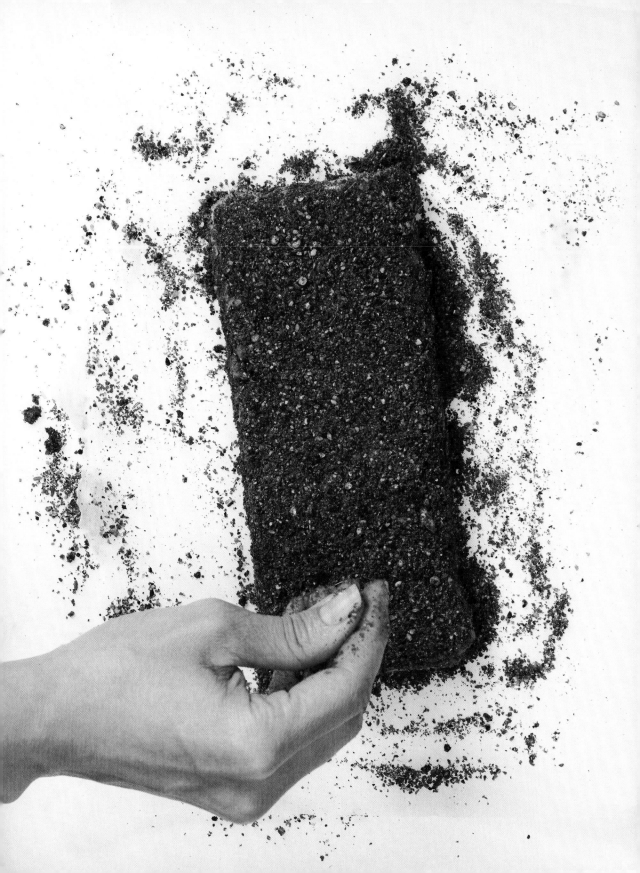

ROASTED LEMON PEPPER CHICKPEAS

Makes 4 cups

2 (14-ounce) cans chickpeas, drained but not rinsed

2 tablespoons lemon juice

½ teaspoon grated lemon zest

3 tablespoons olive oil

1 teaspoon kosher salt

½ teaspoon ground black pepper

Seasoned and roasted to crunchy perfection, hardworking chickpeas add a welcome pop of texture and nutrition to any salad. Toss together a few batches of chickpeas while prepping some dressings and spinning your greens, and suddenly you're ready for a week of hearty salads.

Chickpeas also reveal their different personalities, depending on how long you choose to roast the beans. At around 25 minutes, they are crisp on the outside and soft in the middle; once cooled, they will become chewy. Keep on roasting for another 10 to 12 minutes and the chickpeas dry out substantially and have a nutlike crunch and rich roasted flavor. Keep a watchful eye at this point to make sure they don't burn. Like oven-roasted nuts, chickpeas will continue to brown for a bit even after they're removed from the oven.

Preheat the oven to 375°F. Line a large rimmed baking sheet, or two smaller rimmed baking sheets, with parchment paper for speedy cleanup.

Drain the chickpeas well, and shake to remove any excess canned liquid. No need to rinse; we'll take advantage of the coating of protein-loaded chickpea water encasing the beans to bake in a hearty coating. Transfer the beans to a mixing bowl, add the remaining ingredients, and stir to coat. Spread in a single layer on the baking sheet.

Roast for 20 to 25 minutes, stirring occasionally, for softer chickpeas, or for 35 to 40 minutes for crunchier chickpeas. But watch closely and be careful not to burn the chickpeas at this longer roasting stage. Remove from the oven promptly once they are well browned to prevent burning. Cool completely if not using right away and store in a loosely covered container. Store in the refrigerator and use within 3 days for the best flavor.

variation

Choose your "flavorite" chickpea: Add *one* of the following spice blends or spice combos to create roasted crunchy chickpeas to suit any number of cuisines and salads:

1½ teaspoons ras el hanout (amazing with Middle Eastern—and Moroccan-inspired salads)

1½ teaspoons curry powder

1½ teaspoons garam masala (my favorite with Indian salads)

½ teaspoon each oregano, thyme, basil

1½ teaspoons herbes de Provence

SALT-AND-PEPPER FRIED WHITE BEANS

Makes 2 cups

2 tablespoons olive oil

1 (14-ounce) can white beans, drained, rinsed, and patted dry

2 tablespoons lemon juice, divided

1 garlic clove, minced

Lots of freshly ground black pepper and sea salt, to taste

1 tablespoon nutritional yeast

Chewy and crisp on the outside, and creamy in the center, gently pan-fried white beans are great with bitter greens or as a side dish to any leafy salad. Butter beans are best, but softer cannellini beans can work in flash. A sneakily simple recipe but a tasty alternative to tofu on salads.

Heat a 10-inch cast-iron skillet over medium-high heat for 2 minutes. Drizzle the oil in the pan, then add the beans and sprinkle with half of the lemon juice. Fry the beans for 2 minutes, flipping them occasionally.

Sprinkle with the remaining lemon juice and garlic. Fry for another 1 to 2 minutes, flipping occasionally.

Sprinkle the beans with plenty of freshly cracked pepper, a little salt, and the nutritional yeast. Toss a few times in the pan and serve hot. These are especially great if layered while hot directly on greens to slightly wilt and soften them up. For the best flavor, eat immediately, but if you must, store chilled in a tightly covered container and reheat within 2 days.

SALAD RICE, DRESSED LENTILS, OR OTHER GRAINS OR BEANS

Simply seasoned, wholesome lentils, beans, and whole grains can be the backbone of nearly any salad. Have a few containers of freshly prepared lentils and grains ready to go on Sunday, and super-healthy weekday lunches and dinners practically make themselves.

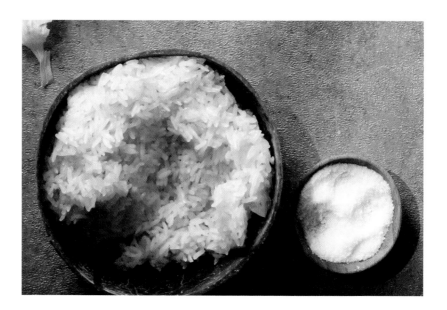

DRESSED LENTILS

Makes 3 cups lentils

1½ cups dark green lentils, black beluga lentils, or French (de Puy) lentils

1 bay leaf

2 garlic cloves, unpeeled and gently crushed

1½ teaspoons kosher salt

1 tablespoon olive oil

1 tablespoon white wine vinegar

If you're going to put lentils in salad (you should—they're cheap, tasty, and loaded with plant-based protein and fiber), you can't go with just any lentil. Go for firm green, black, or French lentils that stay bouncy and toothsome in salads. The most popular of these varieties are dark-green speckled French (de Puy) and beluga lentils, which are smaller lentils with a rounder shape that stay firm and assertive when cooked. A generous amount of kosher salt in the cooking water binds lots of flavor into these little firm lentils, and just a touch of oil and vinegar gives them a light seasoning making them ready for any salad you toss 'em at.

Combine the lentils, 3 cups of water, bay leaf, garlic, and salt in a large saucepan and bring to a rapid boil over high heat. Boil for 2 minutes, stir, then reduce the heat to low and partially cover. Simmer for 40 minutes, or until the lentils are al dente—firm but tender to the bite. Remove and discard the bay leaf and garlic cloves. Drain and rinse with cool water to stop cooking. Transfer to a mixing bowl and toss with the oil and vinegar. Use the lentils in salads right away, or if chilled in an airtight container, allow them to warm slightly before adding to salads. Use within 3 days for the best flavor.

SALAD RICE

Makes 3 cups

1 cup short-grain brown rice, forbidden rice, or red Bhutan rice

½ teaspoon kosher salt

2 teaspoons rice vinegar

With so many great whole grains in the world, it's tempting to overlook good old-fashioned whole-grain rice in salads. Whole-grain rice, once cooled to room temperature, has a nutty, chewy, appealing texture that stands up to assertive dressings, greens, and hearty toppings.

Short-grain brown rice is still my rice of choice for hearty, wholesome salads. The firm, chewy texture and nutty flavor go well with Asian-inspired salads and other combinations of flavors. While the classic ratio for short-grain brown rice is 1:2 rice to water, I prefer just a little less water for fully cooked rice that's slightly drier and firmer for salad.

In a small saucepan, combine the rice, 1¾ cups of water, and salt. Bring to a rolling boil over high heat for 3 minutes, stir the rice once, and cover. Reduce the heat to low and simmer for 35 to 40 minutes, or until all the liquid is absorbed and the rice is tender. Turn off the heat and keep the rice covered for 5 minutes, then transfer the rice to a mixing bowl. Sprinkle with the vinegar. Stir with a fork to separate the clumps and cool the rice. Cool for about 20 minutes, but try to dress the rice while it's still slightly warm.

HOMEMADE BEANS

Makes 5 to 6 cups of cooked beans, with 2 to 3 cups of bean broth

1 pound dry beans, such as black beans, chickpeas, limas, or most any common bean

1 teaspoon kosher salt

1 bay leaf

3-inch strip konbu (dried kelp strips) (optional)

Canned beans rescue countless everyday meals, but occasionally making dry beans from scratch has added rewards: extreme thrift, more variety, and sublimely tasty beans. Homemade beans only have a few rules: some planning ahead, salt, and no added acids until tender.

Time: Poorly cooked beans are typically underdone (rather than overcooked). Keep simmering beans until they are easy to crush with your tongue on the roof of your mouth and the centers are creamy and starchy (like a boiled potato) rather than hard, overly grainy, or crunchy.

Salt: A generous portion of salt to cooking water helps tenderize beans and infuses them with flavor all the way through.

Lastly, dry beans are cooked without the addition of acidic food (tomatoes, vinegar, peppers, beer/wine, citrus juices). Add these flavorful ingredients only after beans are thoroughly cooked and completely tender.

Sort the beans and remove any stones, debris, or broken or off-looking beans. The easiest way to do this is to spread the beans on a dinner plate. Transfer the beans to a large bowl and cover with at least 3 inches of cold water and soak overnight or 8 hours.

Drain the soaking liquid from the beans, rinse the beans, and pour into a large soup pot with a lid. Add about 5 cups of water or enough to cover the beans by about 4 inches. Stir in the salt, bay leaf, and konbu, if using. Cover the pot and bring to a boil over high heat. Skim and discard any foam that rises to the top as it boils. Reduce the heat to low, cover the pot, and simmer for 2 to 2½ hours until done. Perfectly cooked beans should be very soft with a tender interior and soft exterior and will mash easily when pressed with your tongue onto the roof of your mouth.

Store the cooked beans in airtight containers in their cooking liquid. Cool completely before storing the beans, and use within 4 days. You can also freeze the beans; store in 2-cup portions for easy thawing.

QUINOA FOR SALAD

About 3 cups

1 cup quinoa
(white, red, black,
or a blend)

½ teaspoon
kosher salt

Quinoa is a nutritious and familiar addition to salads these days. I don't rely on it nearly as much as I used to. I prefer red quinoa over white, but I often like to blend two or more shades of quinoa for a confetti effect. When I do prepare quinoa, I veer a little sideways from the instructions on the package and use a little less water and dry toast the grain before cooking for a boost of flavor.

Rinse the quinoa with cold running water in a fine-mesh strainer to remove the bitter saponins that naturally cover the seeds. Dump the quinoa into a 2-quart pot, and stirring occasionally over medium heat, toast the quinoa until dry and just starting to smell roasted, about 3 to 4 minutes. Stir in 1¾ cups of water (it will sputter at first), add the salt, increase the heat to high, and bring to a rolling boil. Stir a few times, reduce the heat to low, and cover. Cook for 20 minutes, or until the water has been absorbed and the quinoa grains are tender. Remove from the heat and fluff with a fork. Use in recipes or store, covered in the fridge, up to 3 days. Cooked quinoa is easy to freeze and use later: store 1-cup servings in small zip-top plastic bags, patting the bags flat, and freeze until firm. Use within 3 months. To thaw, leave in the fridge overnight or on the counter for 20 minutes, breaking up the bag as it warms up.

NUTTY, CHEESY, CRUNCHY TOPPINGS

uts have long been the ideal ingredient of choice to create cheese-like toppings. Here a few options for ready-to-sprinkle crunchy, fatty, salty flourishes that liven up any salad.

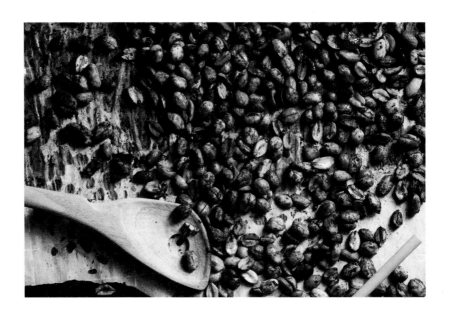

TOASTED SUN AND PEPITA PARM

Makes 1 cup

½ cup pepitas

½ cup raw shelled sunflower seeds

3 tablespoons nutritional yeast

2 teaspoons white miso

½ teaspoon kosher salt

Fatty, salty, tangy: This medley of ground-up seeds, nutritional yeast, miso, and salt steps in for grated hard cheese on salads and checks all the right boxes. It's also perfect and delicious right out of the food processor, but the extra step of gently roasting in the oven coaxes out more toasted, nutty notes.

In a blender or mini food processor, pulse together the pepitas and sunflower seeds into coarse crumbs. Add the nutritional yeast and the miso; break up the miso into smaller bits before pulsing. Add the salt and pulse until mixture is evenly the texture of coarse bread crumbs.

The parm is ready to eat as is, but for a richer, deeper flavor, toast it! Preheat the oven to 325°F. On a baking sheet lined with parchment paper, or a shallow casserole dish, spread in a thin layer. Roast the parm, stirring occasionally, until lightly toasted and fragrant. Remove promptly once the parm is pale golden brown (take care not to over-brown or it will become bitter), and cool completely on the sheet until storing in an airtight container in the fridge. Keep chilled until ready to use.

7-SPICE PEANUTS

Makes 2 cups

⅓ cup apple cider vinegar or umeboshi plum vinegar

1 tablespoon dark or light agave nectar

1 teaspoon Chinese 5-spice powder

½ teaspoon smoked hot paprika (or ½ teaspoon paprika + ¼ teaspoon cayenne pepper)

½ teaspoon chipotle pepper powder

1 teaspoon kosher salt

2 cups unsalted peanuts

A drenching of fruity apple cider vinegar makes these tangy, spicy, salty peanuts right at home poured by the handful on so many salads, and also a snack with hot green tea or a cold beer. Depending on where you live, truly raw peanuts can be hard to come by. Fortunately, easier-to-score lightly roasted, unsalted peanuts work just as well.

In a mixing bowl, whisk together the vinegar, agave, spices, and salt. Stir in the peanuts and marinate for 20 minutes, stirring occasionally. Preheat the oven to 325°F and line a large baking sheet with parchment paper or nonstick foil.

Spread the peanuts in a single layer over the parchment paper and drizzle any excess marinade over the peanuts. Roast for about 20 to 25 minutes, stirring occasionally, until the peanuts are dry and shiny. Cool completely on the sheet and store in a tightly covered container in a cool, dark place, and do try to eat some on a salad and not just by the handful.

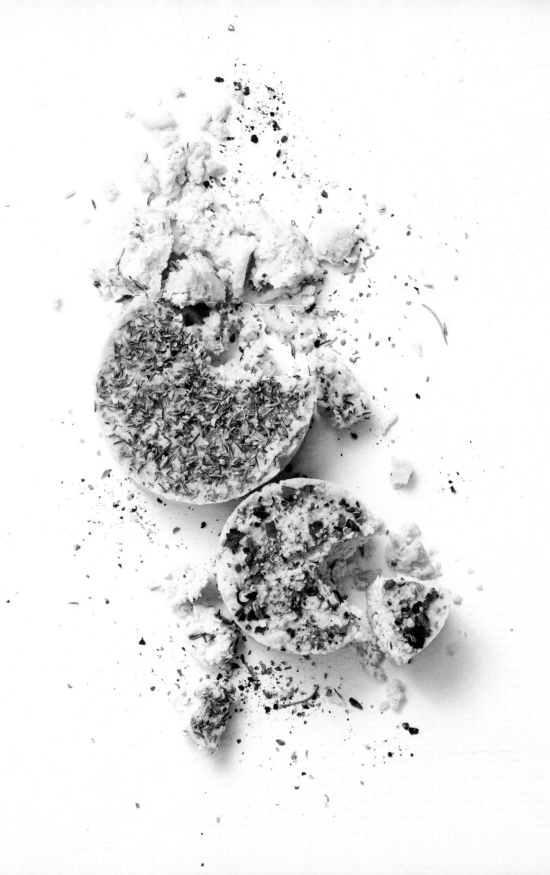

CRUMBLY, SALTY ALMOND CHEESE

Makes 2 (4-inch-round) cheeses

1 cup sliced, blanched almonds

½ cup unroasted cashew pieces

1 vegan probiotic powder capsule

1¼ teaspoons kosher salt

1 teaspoon lemon juice

1 tablespoon nutritional yeast

OPTIONAL COATINGS

2 teaspoons dried oregano, dried thyme, or minced chives

A few healthy twists of pink salt, flaky sea salt, or coarsely ground black pepper

1 tablespoon olive oil

Hearty salads still get major tasty benefits from just a sprinkle of something sharp, tangy, salty, and a little fatty. In a world with better off-the-shelf vegan cheese options every day, I still enjoy dabbling in the occasional DIY vegan cheese project. For those times when you're hungry for a versatile dairy-free "salad cheese" that's kinda like feta, Mexican cotija (or one of many Latin American soft, semi-fresh, and pleasingly salty cheeses), or reminiscent of goat cheese, try your hand at this humble fermented nut cheese. It has a flavor that ranges from sharp to mildly tangy (depending on how long you ferment it) and is assertively salty with a grainy texture, making it fine for breaking apart the little wheels and crumbling on salads, soups, and other good things we like to eat.

This cheese needs a few introverted days of fermenting to cultivate that tangy flavor profile, so plan accordingly. By far, the cleanest and easiest means to ferment nut cheese is scooping out the contents of a vegan probiotic capsule. The flavor results are consistent, and at the end of the day (if you don't bake your cheese), you have a nice little treat loaded with lots of gut-healthy microbes.

Ideally, this cheese is made with a dehydrator; the steady warm temperature and low humidity is perfect for letting the microbes do their work. If you don't have your own, visit your raw foodie friend and ask them if they can babysit your cheese in their dehydrator. A final drying out in a dehydrator (or baking at a low temperature) is essential to help firm up the cheese. (Don't worry if you don't have a dehydrator. See tip Faking It by Baking It, page 115.)

Continued

In a small container, combine the almonds and cashews. Cover with about 2 inches of room-temperature water and soak for 2 hours, or overnight in the fridge.

Drain the nuts and purée in a food processor into a gritty paste. Add ¼ cup of water, then gently open up the probiotic capsule and pour the contents into the nut mixture. Pulse a few more times, scraping down the sides of the processor bowl, until the mixture is a gritty paste.

Cut a piece of cheesecloth about 14 inches wide, and grab a small glass or ceramic bowl (a typical cereal bowl is fine) about 5 inches wide. Use a rubber spatula to scoop out every last bit of the nut mixture into the bowl and smooth it down to a level surface. Lay the cheesecloth over the bowl and secure it with a rubber band around the edge. Set the cheese in the dehydrator for 12 hours at 115°F (see tip if you don't have a dehydrator).

After about 12 hours, the soon-to-be cheese should have a mild, tangy aroma. Peel away the cheesecloth (don't discard). Stir in the salt, lemon juice, and nutritional yeast, and use a silicone spatula to mix thoroughly. Divide the mixture in half.

To help shape a perfectly round cheese, use two 3-inch-wide biscuit cutters.

Cut two more squares of cheesecloth, and layer the older pieces on top of the new pieces (for two stacks of cloth). Place a biscuit cutter in the center of each cloth stack. Use a spoon or rubber spatula to firmly pack half of the nut mixture into each cutter form. Smooth the tops of each cheese evenly and neatly. Move the cheeses to the freezer to firm up for an hour. When each cheese is firm to the touch, remove from the freezer. Carefully slide away each biscuit cutter. Sprinkle the tops of the cheeses with dried herbs, salt and pepper, or olive oil, if desired.

Wrap both cheeses with a double layer of cheesecloth (you can still use that same cheesecloth from earlier). Move to mesh dehydrator sheets and dehydrate for 20 to 30 hours at 115°F or up to 145°F until cheese is very firm and has a dry, crusty exterior. Loosely cover the cheeses and chill thoroughly until ready to use. Stored them in the fridge in a container with a loose-fitting lid. This DIY nut cheese will stay fresh and continue to develop flavor for up to a month.

Tip

FAKING IT BY BAKING IT

The first fermentation stage of the cheese mixture can be done, with a little experimentation, without a dehydrator. Similar to homemade yogurt, try packing the mixture into a thermos, wrapping it with towels, and setting in a draft-free, warm place in your home. Some of the best places can be next to (but not on top of) heating units, on top of the fridge, or even overnight in an oven (which, of course, is turned off and not used).

The second firming/drying stage of this cheese can also be faked via baking. While most or all of the probiotic bacteria will be eliminated by baking,

if you don't have a dehydrator, this is the other option to achieve a firm cheese with a dry exterior and firmer interior.

After the cheese has been shaped and frozen firm, remove from the mold and transfer to a ceramic or glass baking pan. Brush the cheese generously with olive oil and bake in a preheated oven for 300°F for about 30 minutes. A pale golden crust should form around the cheese. Remove from the oven to cool for about 10 minutes, then loosely cover and chill for 3 to 4 hours until completely cold and firm.

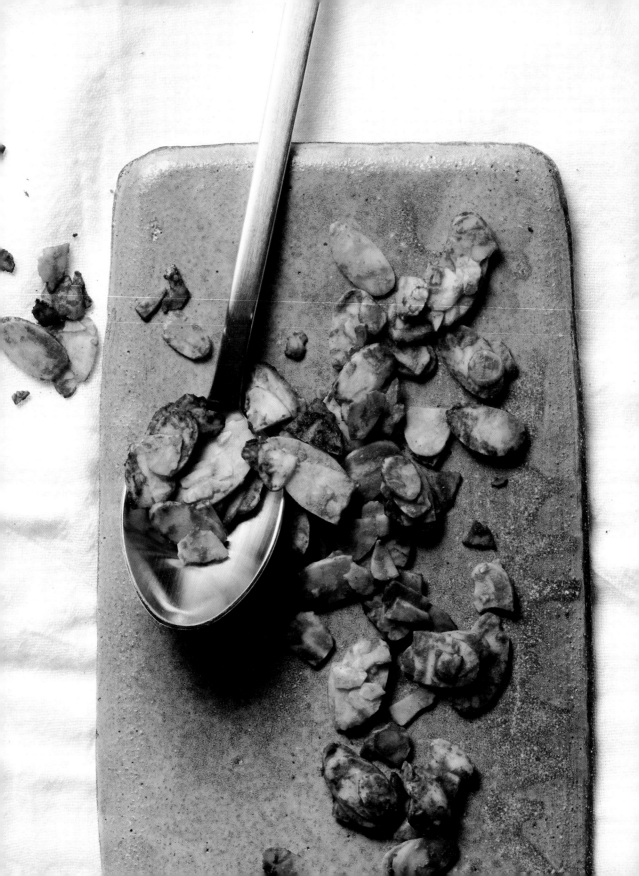

CRISPY, CHEESY ALMOND CRUNCH

Makes 1 cup

2 tablespoons lemon juice

2 tablespoons nutritional yeast

2 teaspoons white miso

½ teaspoon sweet paprika

½ teaspoon turmeric

½ teaspoon salt

⅛ teaspoon cayenne pepper

1 cup blanched, sliced almonds, roughly chopped

Crispy, golden, nibbly almond chips with Cheddar-like notes taste not unlike those neon-yellow fish-shaped crackers. They're clever and fun dancing atop salads that have kid-friendly stuff like apples or grapes, or those especially serious adult ones with a lot of kale.

In a small bowl, whisk together all the ingredients except the almonds into a paste. Fold in the almonds and stir to completely cover the almonds with the paste. Preheat the oven to 325°F and line a baking sheet with parchment paper. Spread the coated almonds in a thin layer over paper and bake for 10 to 12 minutes, stirring occasionally. Roast until the almonds look dry and are toasted on the edge. Watch carefully while roasting and promptly remove from the oven if they get too dark to prevent burning. When completely cool, store in a tightly covered container and use within 2 weeks.

NUT-FREE, SOY-FREE CHEESY SUNFLOWER CRUNCH

Makes 1 cup

2 tablespoons lemon juice

2 tablespoons nutritional yeast

2 teaspoons chickpea miso

½ teaspoon sweet paprika

½ teaspoon salt

¼ teaspoon cayenne pepper

1 cup raw sunflower seeds, roughly chopped

Sunflower seeds replace almonds to make a salad topper and an excellent snack too; tuck into a small container, throw in your backpack, and nibble hiking the Appalachian Trail while contemplating all the work lunchtime salads you're not eating (or just enjoy not being at your desk).

In a mixing bowl, combine all the ingredients, except the seeds, into a creamy paste. Stir in the seeds, taking care to coat all the seeds with paste. Marinate for 30 minutes. Preheat the oven to 325°F and line a baking sheet with parchment paper. Spread the coated seeds in a thin layer over paper and bake for 10 to 12 minutes, stirring occasionally. Roast until the seeds look dry and are toasted. Promptly remove from the oven if they get too dark to prevent burning. When completely cool, store in a tightly covered container and use within 2 weeks.

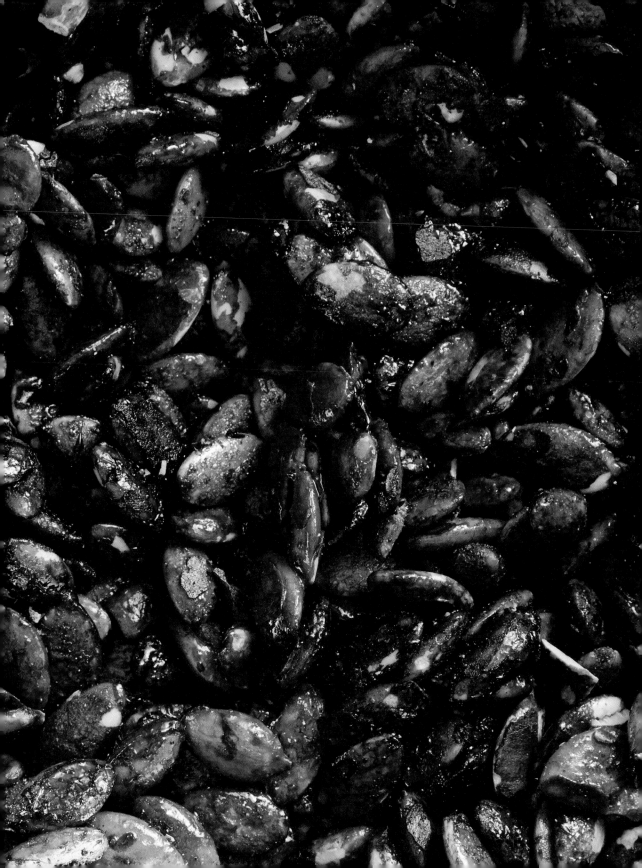

BACON CRUNCH NUTS AND SEEDS

Makes 2 cups

2 cups pepitas

¼ cup maple syrup or amber agave nectar

2 tablespoons tamari

1 teaspoon liquid smoke

½ teaspoon kosher salt

Pinch hot smoked paprika or cayenne pepper and sweet smoked paprika

Sweet-salty-smoky oven-roasted nuts and seeds are good enough to eat by the handful and great enough for virtually any salad. Use the freshest seeds or nuts you can find and make a double batch if you can. Pepitas, if you're unfamiliar, are shelled pumpkin seeds. Loaded with protein and zinc and so good for you, they're a great alternative to nuts, relatively cheap, and ideal crunchy salad toppings. No pepitas? No problem. Sunflower seeds are also perfect here (you can even try a 50/50 blend). Or for a substantial twist, use hazelnuts or pecans (see variations).

Preheat the oven to 325°F and line a large rimmed baking sheet with parchment paper. Lightly spray the paper with olive oil baking spray, or brush with a little oil. In a mixing bowl, combine all the ingredients together. Stir aggressively to thoroughly coat all the seeds. Spread the seeds in an even, thin layer over the parchment paper.

Bake for 20 to 25 minutes, stirring occasionally. Make sure to stir the seeds on the edges of the sheet toward the center, as these tend to brown much faster than the seeds in the middle of the sheet. Watch carefully toward the end of the roast to prevent overbaking.

Remove from the oven promptly once they are golden brown and shiny. Cool completely on the sheet before storing in an airtight container. Use within 2 weeks for the best flavor, if they even last longer than a few days.

variation

BACON CRUNCH HAZELNUTS

My favorite variation of this recipe, made just as often as the original. Replace the pepitas with 2 cups roughly chopped hazelnuts. If using whole, use unpeeled hazelnuts. You may need to increase the roasting time another 5 minutes.

BACON CRUNCH PECANS

Replace the pepitas with 2 cups of whole pecan halves. Increase the roasting time another 5 to 10 minutes as needed until pecans are lightly browned, but watch carefully to prevent burning.

SWEET AND SALTY PECANS

Leave out the liquid smoke for simply sweet and savory glazed pecans; roast as described for Bacon Crunch Pecans.

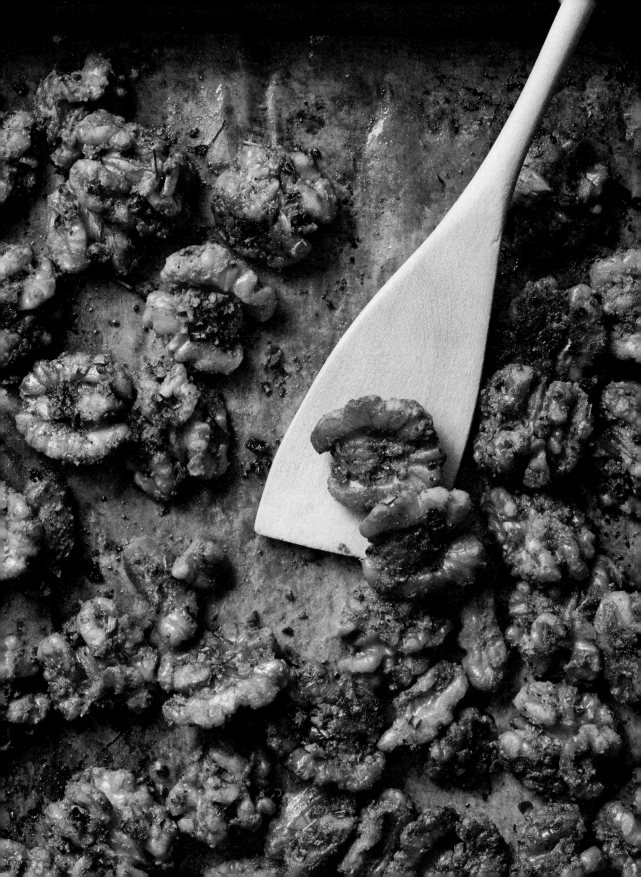

CAESAR WALNUTS

Makes about 2 cups

2 tablespoons capers, drained

2 garlic cloves, peeled

1 teaspoon garlic powder

1½ teaspoons kosher salt

1 teaspoon mustard powder

½ teaspoon ground black pepper

2 tablespoons nutritional yeast

2 tablespoons lemon juice

6 ounces (about 2 cups) walnut halves

Preheat the oven to 300°F and line a baking sheet with aluminum foil or parchment paper.

Zesty, salty, savory, crunchy, these roasty walnut halves basically are concentrated Caesar dressing bombs that bring salad flavors to anything, including more Caesar to your average Caesar salad. A punch of fresh garlic and garlic powder, along with dependable cheesy flavor from nutritional yeast, makes these dreamy salad toppers and party nibbles. Just try not to eat the entire serving standing at the kitchen counter, and save some for scattering on top of salads.

In a mini food processor, pulse together all the ingredients except the walnuts for 30 seconds into a rough paste, or pound in a mortar and pestle. Use a rubber spatula to scoop the paste into a mixing bowl, add the walnuts, and vigorously stir to coat the walnuts with the paste. Or like some of my testers, use your fingers to rub the paste into the walnuts.

Spread in a single layer on the foil and roast the nuts for 10 to 12 minutes. Watch carefully! Oven-roasted nuts love to sprint from golden to burned almost instantly; once the nuts have achieved a nice tan, promptly remove from the oven, as they will continue to toast for another 30 seconds or so until cooled. Cool completely and store in the fridge in an airtight container. Gobble up within a week for the best flavor.

CRISPY, CHEWY VEGGIE TOPPINGS

More vegetables on TOP of the salad? Yes! Seasoned and thoughtfully roasted or seared or even pickled mushrooms, roots, and onions are a brilliant way to add intense flavor and texture to any salad or soup. Especially in the instance of vegetable "bacons," they may even become the best part of the whole dish.

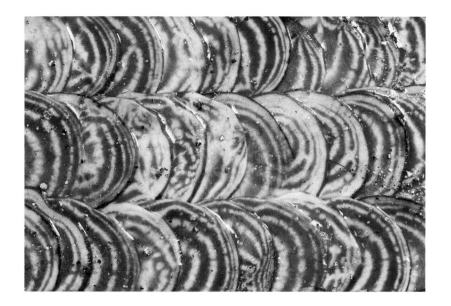

MAPLE MUSHROOM BACON

Makes 1 generous cup

8 ounces shiitake, maitake, or similar fleshy edible mushroom

2 tablespoons tamari

2 tablespoons pure maple syrup

2 tablespoons extra-virgin olive oil

1 teaspoon balsamic vinegar

¼ teaspoon chipotle powder

¼ teaspoon kosher salt

There's nothing quite like mushroom bacon. Earthy and smoky, the slippery, chewy texture of roasted candied mushrooms mimics the mouthfeel of fatty bacon, without being either. Shiitake, long-reigning champ of homemade mushroom bacon, is naturally suited for the job; shiitakes are a relatively cheap, "wild" (yet cultivated) mushroom with a rich flavor unlike pedestrian white button supermarket 'shrooms.

But there is a bacony world beyond shiitakes! I encourage you to branch out to include maitake (hen of the woods), oyster, or unusual pioppino or king trumpet. Maitake makes wonderful mushroom bacon. This petal-like mushroom tears easily for dense, chewy bites of bacon, and thinly sliced jumbo portobellos, the overgrown rustic cousin of the everyday brown supermarket mushroom, make appealing strips of deep, dark veggie bacon.

Remove the stems from the shiitakes or portabellos. If using portabellos, use a small spoon to scrape away and discard the dark gills from underneath the caps (they don't taste very good). Slice into pieces no thicker than ¼ inch thick. If using maitake mushrooms, slice away any very tough "root" bases and tear the mushrooms into ½-inch-wide strips. In a large bowl, whisk together the remaining ingredients for the marinade.

Add the mushrooms and toss for at least a minute; thoroughly coat the mushrooms with the marinade. Cover and marinate for 20 minutes. While the mushrooms are marinating, preheat the oven to 350°F and line a large baking sheet with parchment paper.

Continued

Spread the mushrooms in a single layer. Roast for 20 minutes, stirring every 6 to 8 minutes, or until the mushrooms are crisp on the ends and a little chewy in the center; the mushroom slices will reduce by over half or more. Most mushrooms are 92 percent water!

Remove from the oven promptly to avoid burning and cool completely before storing in an airtight container. Keep chilled until ready to use, and enjoy within a week for the best flavor.

variation

This recipe also makes great mushroom jerky! Simply marinate the mushrooms overnight, then spread on solid dehydrator sheets and dry for 18 to 24 hours or as directed in your dehydrator instructions.

ROOT BACON

Makes about ½ pound

1 pound parsnips or carrots (rainbow carrots are excellent here)

¼ cup agave nectar

1 tablespoon apple cider vinegar

2 tablespoons olive oil

2 teaspoons smoked paprika

½ teaspoon liquid smoke

½ teaspoon salt

Crispy, savory, smoky strips made from root veggies—obvious? Yes. Delicious? Yes. Parsnips and carrots are sweet, and they play well with salt, syrups, and sweet spices like paprika. The process for making both veggie root bacons is exactly the same, but the results are different!

Roasted uncovered, parsnips have an earthy aroma and a tender, chewy texture. Sweet, colorful carrots get even sweeter and get a little crispy on the edges. Different root bacons are fun to serve together, so I usually make ½ pound of each (or a bunch of different-colored carrot bacons) and divide the marinade among the bowls. But they are definitely better if you prepare each batch in a separate bowl (especially since the juices of most any color carrot—purple, red, orange, multihued—will stain the spongy flesh of the white parsnips).

Preheat the oven to 325°F. Line two large baking sheets with parchment paper and liberally brush or spray with cooking oil. Scrub the roots well and pat dry. No need to peel, as we'll be slicing them so thin the skin will never be noticed.

Use a mandoline (preferably a Japanese one that allows very fine-tuning of the slices), and slice each root lengthwise into strips about ¹/₁₆ of an inch thick or as thin as possible. These slices should be papery thin.

In a large mixing bowl, whisk together the remaining marinade ingredients. Add the root slices and toss (hands are best for this maneuver) and rub each piece with the marinade to thoroughly coat every slice. Lay each vegetable slice on the sheet; don't overlap the slices. It's

Continued

okay if some of the edges occasionally touch, but you will get better results if each piece has some space to allow it to roast, rather than steam, while in the oven.

Slide each sheet into the oven and roast for about 10 minutes. At 10 minutes, remove the sheet and flip over each strip. Rotate the sheets and put them back into the oven and roast for another 4 to 6 minutes, or until the edges are crisp and centers are tender. Watch carefully, as root bacon can burn easily.

Root vegetable bacon is best when hot and crisp, but leftovers can be chilled, tightly covered, for up to 2 days. For best results, reheat the cold root bacon in the oven at 350°F for 8 to 10 minutes, flipping halfway through, until crisped on the edges.

tip

Parchment paper is essential for fast and easy cleanup. These paper-thin vegetable strips are delicate and become even easier to rip once they are roasted, so the nonstick properties of oiled parchment paper will help make lifting the strips easy and tear-free.

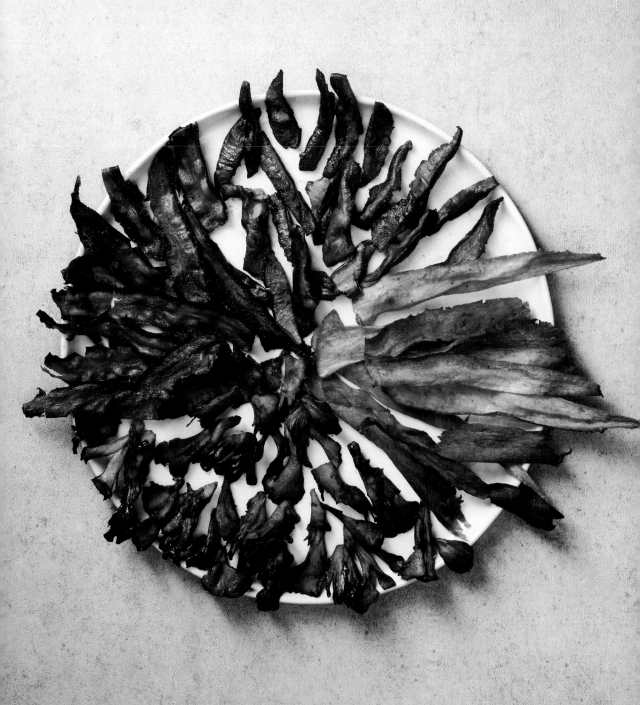

PASTRAMI CARROTS

Makes 1 pound of roasted carrots, for 3 to 4 servings

3 tablespoons olive oil, plus additional for oiling the dish

1½ pounds carrots

Pastrami spice mix from Whole-Loaf Blackened Tempeh Pastrami recipe (page 97)

1 tablespoon organic brown sugar

Tender, toothsome, and brimming with flavor, these sausage-like roasted carrots are another way to enjoy that kicking pastrami spice rub. They are excellent on any salad but exceptional just served with a dollop of Tahini Mayo (page 43) or a drizzle of Tahini French Dressing (page 45) and a handful of greens.

Preheat the oven to 375°F and rub the insides of a 10 x 10 x 2-inch or 11 x 7 x 2-inch baking dish generously with oil. Wash and scrub the carrots, pat dry, and trim off any root tops. Slice in half lengthwise any carrots wider than 1½ inches.

In the baking dish, use your fingers or a fork to combine the spice mix, 1 tablespoon oil, and brown sugar. Rub the carrots with a little oil and lay on top of the spice blend. Rub the spice blend into the carrots and pat a thin layer of spices over the carrots (they tend to stick better to the cut sides).

Arrange the carrots in as much of a single layer as possible (some overlap is fine) snugly into the baking dish. Drizzle with the remaining 2 tablespoons of olive oil. Crimp a layer of foil tightly over the dish and roast in the preheated oven for 25 minutes. Remove the foil and continue to roast for another 15 to 20 minutes, or until the carrots are extremely tender (easy to pierce with the tip of a knife) and beautifully browned. Serve hot or room temperature, and enjoy within 3 days.

BEET PROSCIUTTO

Makes about 1 pound, about 3 to 4 servings

1 pound beets, about 2 large beets (3 inches wide), well scrubbed, fine roots removed, ends trimmed

3 tablespoons red wine vinegar

2 teaspoons kosher salt

2 tablespoons organic brown sugar

1 teaspoon smoked sweet paprika

1 teaspoon garlic powder

½ teaspoon ground black pepper

Generous pinch cayenne pepper

¼ cup chickpea liquid (a.k.a. aquafaba, the liquid from about 1 to 2 cans of chickpeas)

Inspired by the phenomenon that is carrot lox (and if you're wondering, the best carrot lox can be found at Orchard Grocery in New York City's Lower East Side)—a similar process that makes roots into faux lox transforms beets to veggie prosciutto. The finished product is a mass of a spiced, salty-sweet, supple strips of beets that function like prosciutto in salads. It's great paired with fatty nut-based cheese, bitter greens, and juicy fruits in salads throughout the year.

For the prettiest beet prosciutto, use the widest parts of the largest beets you can find, about 2½ inches in diameter. Don't peel the beets; the root skin creates a rustic edge for that cured meaty look. And definitely try this with different-colored beets! Red beets create classic deep red slices, golden beet ham is ethereal, and magenta-and-white-ringed Chioggia beets create soft pink rippled root ham that echoes the marbled slices of traditional prosciutto.

Trim any scraggly roots from the beets, and slice off the end of each beet about ½ inch from the root and stem ends. The goal is to start with slices of beets about 1½ inches wide from the center of the beets (save the ends of the beets for other recipes). Use a mandoline to slice the beets paper thin, 1/16 of an inch.

Transfer the beet slices to a mixing bowl and add the vinegar, salt, brown sugar, paprika, garlic powder, black pepper, and cayenne. Toss with your hands and massage the beets; the beets will soften up and release a good deal of juice. Drain away the liquid and transfer the beets to a gallon-sized zip-top plastic bag. Seal the bag, pressing out any excess air. Layer the bag in the bottom of the mixing

Continued

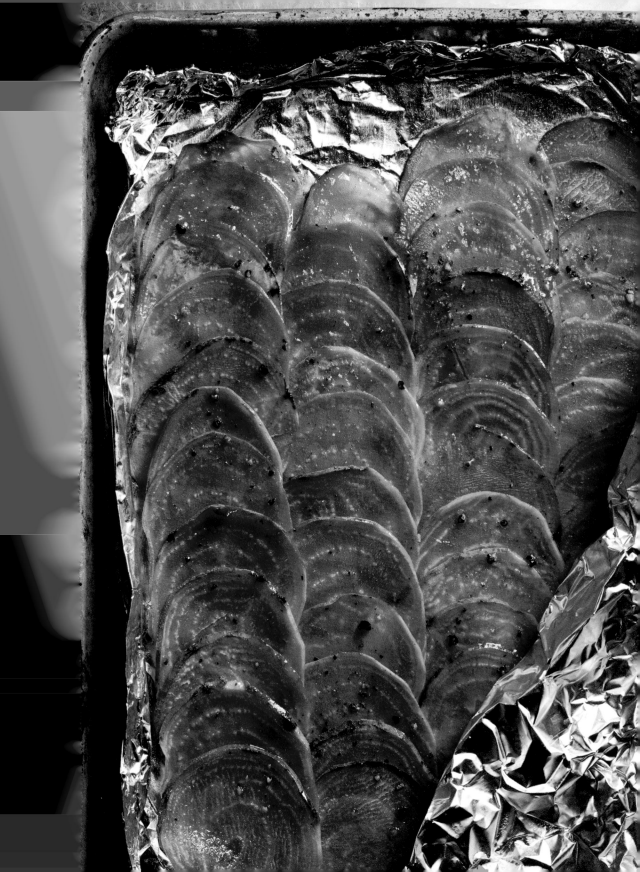

bowl and add a few heavy things on top of the bag. Leave the beets alone to press and marinate for at least 4 hours or overnight in the fridge.

When you're ready to roast the beets, line a large baking sheet with a sheet of foil about 14 inches long, shiny side up. Brush or spray the foil with olive oil. Pour chickpea liquid into a large mixing bowl.

Preheat the oven to 350°F. Drain any excess liquid from the beets. Take a slice of beet and shake to remove excess moisture. Dip the beet slice in the chickpea liquid, shake off the excess liquid, then lay the beet slice flat on the oiled foil about 2 inches from the upper-left-hand corner. Repeat with another slice and arrange on top of the previous slice, leaving about ½ inch of the slice underneath showing. Continue overlapping with the remaining beets, creating a few rows of overlapping beets; the result should be a rough rectangle of overlapping beets, about 12 inches long (see the lovely close-up on page iv of Chioggia beet prosciutto before baking or page 132 of the beet prosciutto after baking). Drizzle any remaining chickpea liquid over the beets.

Cover the top of the foil with another sheet of foil the same size (shiny side down) and crimp the edges of the foil sheets (use those 2 inches of border to crimp tightly) to create a big foil pouch. Bake for 25 minutes; the crimped edges will steam the beets inside and prevent them from drying out. Remove from the oven and leave them covered for 2 minutes, then peel back the foil and cool. Use a spatula to lift the beets off the foil and stack on top of each other in an airtight container. Chill the beet prosciutto thoroughly before serving, and use within 3 days for the best flavor.

PAN-ROASTED CHILE CORN

Makes 2 cups

1 tablespoon extra-virgin olive oil

2 cups fresh or lightly thawed frozen corn kernels (see tip)

1 tablespoon lime juice

2 teaspoons ancho chile powder or chili powder blend

1¼ teaspoons kosher salt

With a touch of olive oil and a cast-iron pan, regular ol' corn turns into blistered, gently charred nibbles perfect for collard greens or kale and anything with avocado. Make the most of fresh corn in the summer, or liven up that lonely bag of frozen corn and add summer vibes to salads and soups all year round.

Heat a cast-iron pan over medium-high heat. Add the oil and corn kernels. Stir occasionally and roast until the corn is just starting to char, about 3 minutes. Sprinkle in the lime juice, chili powder, and salt. Stir-fry the corn for 1 more minute, then transfer to a bowl to cool. Store corn in the refrigerator in an airtight container and use within 2 days for the best flavor.

tip

If using frozen corn, lightly thaw by placing frozen corn in a large metal colander and rinsing with cool water until the corn has thawed slightly. Break up the kernels under the running water to help thaw evenly.

CRISPY LIME-AND-SALT SHALLOTS

Makes about 1½ cups

½ pound (about 4 to 6 large 2-inch-long) shallots

1 cup high-heat canola oil, grape-seed, or rice bran oil

2 tablespoons freshly squeezed lime juice

2 teaspoons kosher salt

Crunchy and sweet, these easy shallots look like flour-dredged fried onion bits but couldn't be any easier. The key to great fried shallots seems counterintuitive: Instead of plunging the shallots in hot oil, sliced shallots are placed in the cold pan, with cold oil, and then heated until the shallots fry and brown. The process helps create beautifully caramelized yet crunchy shallots that, once properly drained and cooled, will remain crisp and fresh-tasting for up to 3 weeks.

Peel the shallots and slice about ⅛ inch thick. Use your fingers to separate the slices into rings. Pour the oil into a wok or stable, steep-sided pot for deep frying. Layer a large dish with a few paper towels or crinkled brown paper, and have handy a long-handled metal mesh skimmer.

Add the shallots and heat the oil over medium-high heat. It will take anywhere from 5 to 8 minutes (or a little more) to get the shallots sizzling. Watch the shallots carefully; they will look rather pale for a few minutes, then rapidly change from golden to dark brown, then to burned. The goal is to rescue the shallots from the oil when they've reached a rich golden brown but are still a few shades removed from burned. Skim out the shallots and spread on the paper. Turn off the heat.

While the shallots are still hot, transfer to a mixing bowl and sprinkle with the lime juice and salt, stirring a few times to coat with the seasonings. Cool the shallots completely before storing in an airtight container, and use within 3 weeks for the best flavor.

Tip

The richly flavored shallot oil can be strained and saved for a savory oil to brush on veggies before grilling.

RED ONION QUICK PICKLE

Makes about 1 cup

½ pound (1 large, about 4 to 5 inches wide) red onion

1 tablespoon lime juice

2 teaspoons organic sugar

1 teaspoon kosher salt

½ teaspoon ancho chile or similar mild chili powder

1 teaspoon black mustard seeds

I've been heaping easy pickled red onions onto meals for years. Originally, this speedy pickle recipe was Mexican or Latin American in spirit, then I recalled a favorite everyday Indian chutney—sweet and hot red chile onion chutney—could be hacked with my go-to recipe. It's not exactly like red onion pickle but a cross between an Indian spicy pickle, a sweet chutney, and something a bit Latino.

Whatever it is, I dollop these juicy, tangy, spicy, crunchy, zesty pink shreds on the Red Lentil Khichdi (page 269), White Bean and Seitan Green Posole (page 273), and many salads in this book. You will find so many great ways to enjoy this incredibly easy everyday pickle!

Peel the onion, slice in half, then use a mandoline to slice the onion into paper-thin shreds. Transfer to a mixing bowl and add the lime juice, sugar, salt, and chili powder. In a small skillet, toast the mustard seeds over high heat just until they pop, then pour into the bowl with the onions.

Use a hand to massage the onions with the spices (wear a glove if sensitive to chiles and onions). Massage for about 2 minutes, or until the onions are very tender. You can enjoy immediately or store chilled until ready to eat. Best if gobbled up within 2 days, and so easy to make you can keep a rotating batch on hand anytime.

CROUTONS AND
TOASTY BITES

Bread and salad together create one of the most satisfying meals on the planet. Croutons, those highly seasoned, cleverly upcycled bits of old bread are the perfect way to indulge without overdoing it and are delicious made with any quality bread (even gluten-free!) or a homemade loaf of delicate vegan cornbread.

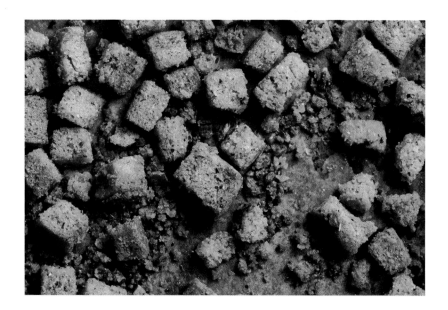

SAVORY COCONUT CHIPS, 3 WAYS

Makes 2 cups

2 cups large flake dried coconut, unsweetened

CHIPOTLE BACON

2 tablespoons tamari

2 tablespoons pure maple syrup

½ teaspoon liquid smoke

½ teaspoon chipotle powder

Generous pinch kosher salt

COCONUT TURMERIC LIME

¼ cup lime juice

1 teaspoon kosher salt

½ teaspoon turmeric powder

¼ teaspoon cayenne pepper

SALT, PEPPER, AND VINEGAR

¼ cup white wine vinegar

1½ teaspoons kosher salt

1 teaspoon cracked black pepper, or cracked multicolored pepper

Big pieces of flavored, roasted coconut are an easy way to add that fatty, crisp something tasty on so many salads. You'll find three flavor variations here, but the possibilities really are endless. Beyond the flavoring, the key is finding exceptionally large pieces of dried coconut; seek out big flakes, such as from Bob's Red Mill, in favor of shredded or tiny pieces of broken coconut. My absolute favorite can be sourced from a trip to an Indian grocery; look for long half-moon crescents of shaved coconut for beautiful and dramatic roasted coconut chips.

Preheat the oven to 325°F and line a large baking sheet with parchment paper. In a mixing bowl, toss together the coconut flakes with the marinade ingredients; gently rub the marinade into the flakes to get everything coated with flavor.

Spread the coconut in a thin layer on the sheet. Roast in the oven for about 15 minutes, stirring occasionally. Watch carefully toward the end to prevent the coconut from burning. The flakes are ready when they are light golden brown and they smell warm and toasty. Promptly remove from the oven and set the baking sheet on a wire rack to cool; the flakes will continue to brown when they are still very hot and straight out of the oven, so it's critical to cool them promptly to avoid burning. Cool completely before storing in an airtight container. Use within a month for the best flavor.

SEEDY GARLIC
BREAD CROUTONS

Makes about 7 cups

10 to 12 ounces
(about 7 to 8 cups
roughly diced)
day-old bread
cubes, preferably
sourdough

4 big fat garlic
cloves, peeled

1 teaspoon
kosher salt

2 tablespoons red
wine vinegar

2 tablespoons
chopped parsley

2 teaspoons dried
oregano

½ cup olive oil

1 tablespoon
shelled hemp
seeds, sesame
seeds, or poppy
seeds

Croutons are amazing—unloved old bread becomes the crunchy jewel that gilds the salad unlike anything else. The catch is for good croutons, one must use good, even great, bread. Rustic whole-grain breads are a staple in my crouton mixes, but sourdough, especially light and tangy San Francisco–style, is my favorite yeasted bread for crowd-pleasing croutons; the texture and flavor simply make excellent croutons ideal for a wide range of salads and scattered on top of soups. Or just eating by the handful.

Preheat the oven to 350°F and line a large baking sheet with parchment paper. Transfer the bread cubes to a large, wide mixing bowl.

In a mortar and pestle, smash together the garlic and salt into a chunky paste. Scoop the paste into a small bowl and whisk in the vinegar, parsley, and oregano. Whisk in the oil, streaming in a little at a time. Add the hemp seeds. Drizzle over the bread cubes and fold into the cubes, coating as much of the bread as possible with the dressing.

Spread the cubes in an even layer over the parchment paper. Bake the cubes for 25 to 30 minutes, stirring occasionally. The croutons are ready when they are golden brown and crisp. Cool in the pan completely before storing in an airtight container. Croutons can resist the ravages of time and—if their container is stored in a cool, dry, dark place—should stay crisp and tasty for up to 6 weeks.

Continued

variation

BASIL PESTO CROUTONS

In the dressing, omit the parsley and oregano. Add ¼ cup chopped, packed basil leaves and add 2 tablespoons nutritional yeast. Whisk together the dressing ingredients and fold into the bread cubes as directed above.

SIMPLE CROUTONS

Super basic and super easy, these use an off-the-shelf herb blend but make your salads look like they were lovingly tended to by a team of next-level food bloggers.

> ½ cup olive oil
>
> 1 tablespoon Italian seasoning blend (especially one with lots of rosemary)
>
> ½ teaspoon salt

Whisk together the dressing ingredients and fold into the bread cubes as directed above.

NAKED TOASTS

When bread is truly flavorful inside *and* out—rustic olive bread, fresh herb bread, a bread studded with lots of nuts and fruits—sometimes nothing is the best seasoning. Tear the stale bread into bite-sized pieces and spread in an even layer on the baking sheet. No dressing required. Toast as directed above. I prefer undressed bread to be a shade or two darker than flavored croutons to bring out the natural flavors of the toast. Cool completely, store in an airtight container, and eat these a little sooner than you would flavored croutons.

NO-OIL CHIA CRUNCH CROUTONS

Makes 6 cups or more

10 to 12 ounces stale bread cubes

2 tablespoons chia seeds

3 tablespoons lemon juice

4 heaping teaspoons dried herb blend (see tip)

1 teaspoon celery seed

1 teaspoon kosher salt

These incredibly light and crunchy bits have against all odds become my favorite croutons. I love my olive oil, but the brightness of these herb-crusted croutons is habit forming.

Stale (a few days old is fine too) bread cubes are essential for making any crouton. Fresh bread will sag and crumble when tossed with seasonings and oil, but it's downright red-alert mission critical in this recipe that the bread be desert-sands dry before adding the marinade. As the water-based marinade contains no oil to speak of, fresh bread will turn to mush within minutes. Giving the bread a pre-toasting makes certain that no hint of moisture remains.

Tip

CHOOSE YOUR HERB BLEND WEAPON

Different herbs for different vibes; croutons can be customized to fit your mood, season, or wardrobe. Off-the-rack blends that are ideal for croutons are:

Italian Herb Blends (featuring oregano, basil, marjoram, etc.)

Herbes de Provence: bright and herbal croutons for leafy salads

Za'atar: savory and tangy, bold herbal flavors that go great with citrus dressings

Preheat the oven to 325°F. While the oven is heating up, spread the stale bread cubes in a single layer on one large (or two smaller) baking sheets and transfer to the oven; as the oven heats, it will lightly toast and crisp up the croutons for 20 minutes.

Meanwhile, whisk together ⅓ cup of water, chia seeds, lemon juice, herb blend, celery seed, and salt. Add the crisp, warm croutons and stir thoroughly to coat everything with marinade. Immediately spread the croutons back onto the baking sheet and put back into the oven.

Bake for 15 to 20 minutes, stirring occasionally. The idea is to get them perfectly crisp and very dry. Remove from the oven and cool completely before storing in zip-top gallon plastic bags or other airtight storage. Like many croutons, these stay tasty for a month or slightly longer.

CHEESY, CRISPY CROUTONS

Makes about 7 cups

10 to 12 ounces (about 7 to 8 cups roughly diced) day-old sourdough bread

3 tablespoons lemon juice

4 teaspoons white miso

2 teaspoons garlic powder

1 teaspoon sweet paprika

½ teaspoon ground turmeric

½ teaspoon kosher salt

¼ cup melted vegan butter

CHEESY CRUSTY SPRINKLE

¼ cup nutritional yeast

¼ cup blanched almond meal (see note)

2 tablespoons melted vegan butter

1½ teaspoons kosher salt

The superheroes of DIY vegan cheese flavors—miso, nutritional yeast, lemon juice—along with tangy sourdough bread create bright and crunchy croutons with a cheesy personality. Sourdough bread is key for making the Cheddar-like notes pop, so be sure to use a punchy rustic loaf in this recipe. Lastly, use the best vegan butter you can get to give these cheesy croutons the richness they (and you) deserve.

Preheat the oven to 350°F and line a large baking sheet with parchment paper. Transfer the bread cubes to a large, wide mixing bowl. In a small mixing bowl, stir together the lemon juice, miso, garlic powder, paprika, turmeric, and salt. Whisk in the melted vegan butter, streaming in a little at a time. Drizzle this mixture over the bread cubes and fold into the cubes, coating as much of the bread as possible with the dressing. In a small separate bowl, combine the nutritional yeast, almond meal, melted vegan butter, and salt. Sprinkle and fold into the cubes.

Spread the cubes in an even layer on the parchment paper. Bake the cubes for 20 to 25 minutes, stirring occasionally. The croutons are ready when they are golden brown and crisp. Cool in the pan completely before storing in an airtight container in a cool, dry, dark place. Use within 4 weeks for the best flavor.

* Make your own almond meal by pulsing ½ cup blanched slivered or sliced almonds in a food processor into fine crumbs. Pulse for a few short bursts, only until the mixture looks crumbly.

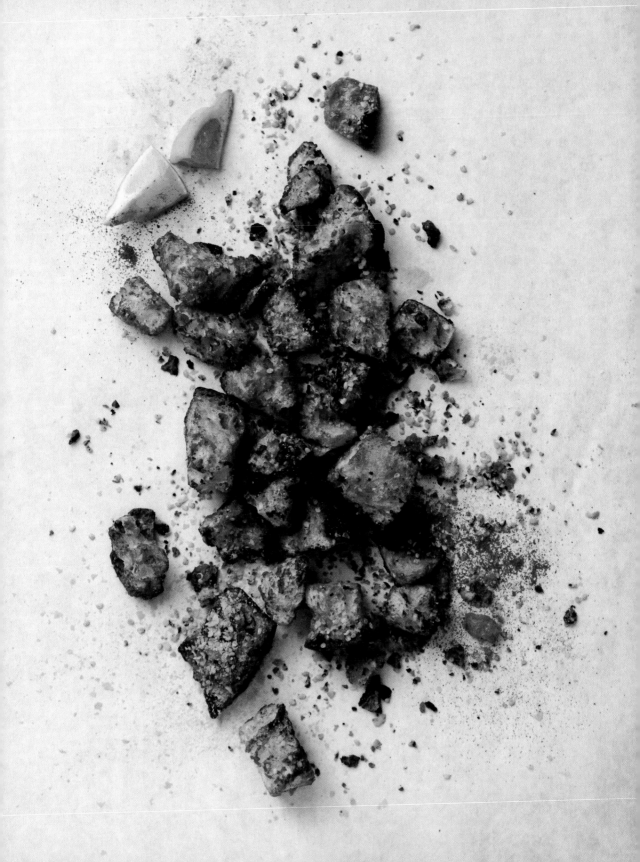

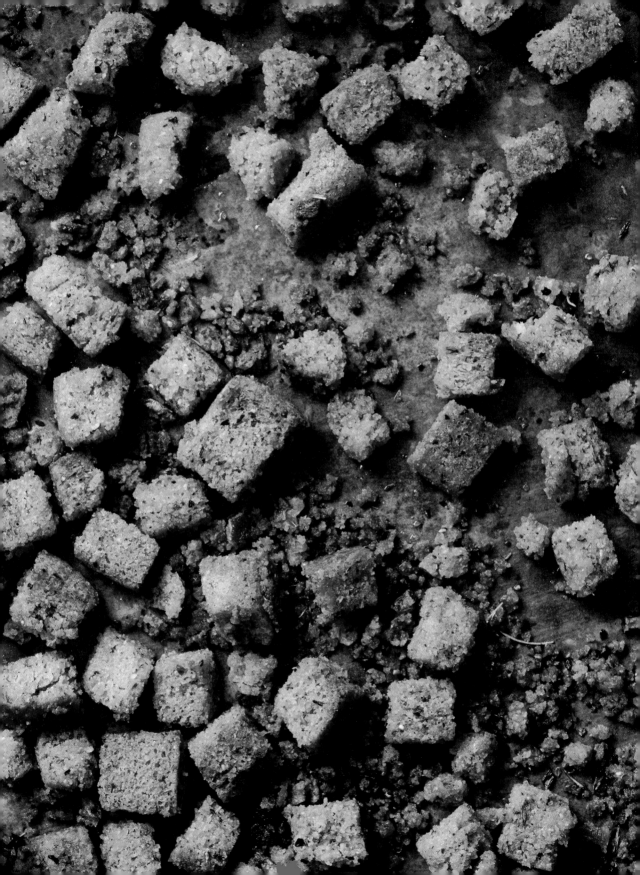

HERBED CORNBREAD CRUNCH

Makes about 4 cups

12 ounces (about 4 cups) day-old vegan cornbread (see Vegan Cornbread Loaf, page 146)

¼ cup olive oil

2 tablespoons apple cider vinegar

1 teaspoon dried thyme

½ teaspoon paprika

½ teaspoon black pepper

½ teaspoon kosher salt

Sweet and golden, cornbread croutons are crunchy and slightly chewy, a substantial twist on croutons made from yeasted wheat breads. These corny babies are essential for collard greens salads or kale anything, and they're perfect on hearty soups. Few bakeries offer vegan cornbread, so I've included a handy recipe for a slightly sweet cornbread baked in a loaf pan, the perfect shape for croutons, toasts, and snacking.

Preheat the oven to 325°F and line a large baking sheet with foil. Dice the day-old cornbread into 1-inch cubes. Spread out onto a baking sheet and gently toast the cubes to dry them out and firm them up, about 20 minutes.

In a large mixing bowl, whisk together the remaining ingredients. Add the croutons and use a rubber spatula to stir the cubes and coat with the marinade, then spread again on the foil in a single layer. Increase oven to 350°F and roast for another 20 to 25 minutes, stirring occasionally, until the cubes are crisp and golden. Remove from the oven and cool completely before using. Store in an airtight container and use within 2 weeks for the best flavor.

VEGAN CORNBREAD LOAF

Makes 1 loaf

2 cups yellow cornmeal

½ cup all-purpose flour

¼ cup organic cane sugar

1½ teaspoons baking powder

½ teaspoon baking soda

1 teaspoon kosher salt

2 cups unsweetened almond milk

1 tablespoon apple cider vinegar

2 tablespoons ground flaxseeds

¼ cup melted refined coconut oil or neutral-tasting vegetable oil

Cornbread in a loaf pan is a convenient shift from the cast-iron pan cornbread experience. The key to making cornbread for croutons (and stuffing too) is to skip baking it in fun things like cast-iron skillets or muffin tins, and opt for a boring, but effective, loaf pan. The thin walls of the loaf pan will create drier, highly desirable crust for your cornbread.

Neat and sliceable, and plenty of surface area for more crust, a loaf of cornbread is great for avocado toast, and then after a day or so, it is exactly the right consistency and shape for slicing into croutons.

Preheat the oven to 350°F and grease an 8½ x 4-inch loaf pan.

Grab a large mixing bowl and stir together the cornmeal, flour, sugar, baking powder, baking soda, and salt. In a separate smaller bowl, whisk together the almond milk, apple cider vinegar, and flaxseeds; set this aside for 2 minutes to help the vinegar curdle the milk and allow the flaxseeds to soak up the liquid and create that wonderful gel that will help bind the loaf together. Whisk in the oil.

Stir the flour mixture and form a well in the center; pour in the liquid ingredients. Use a rubber spatula or dough whisk to stir together the ingredients just enough to moisten the dry ingredients; small lumps in the batter are fine! The key to any tender loaf is to avoid overmixing the batter.

Scoop into the prepared pan and bake for 45 minutes. Insert a sharp knife into the center of the loaf; when the knife emerges clean (a few moist crumbs are fine), it's done! If the batter still seems a little wet, bake for another 10 to 15 minutes. Remove from the oven, let it linger in the pan for 10 minutes, then remove from the pan and cool completely.

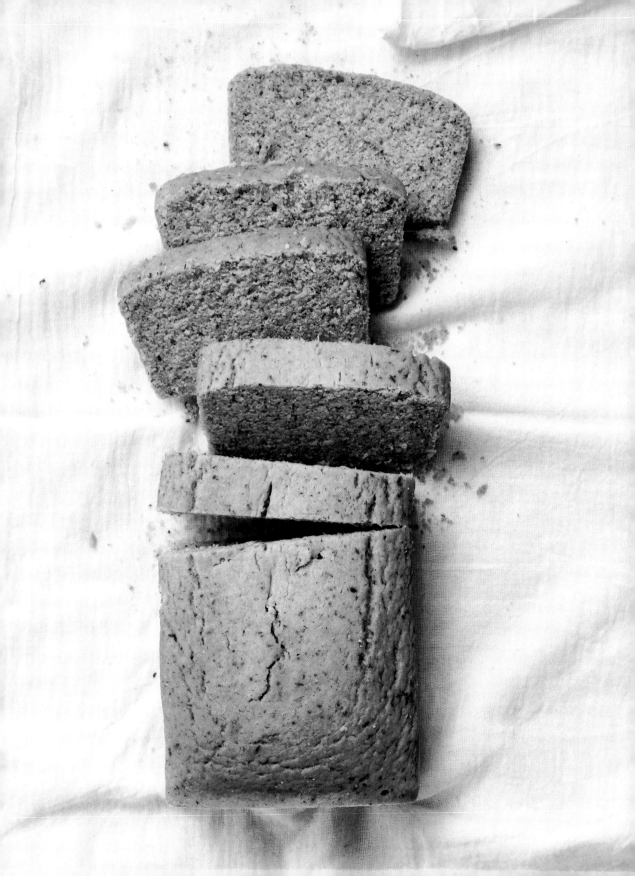

SWEET, SALTY, NUTTY GOMASIO

Makes ¾ cup

½ cup sliced, blanched almonds

¼ cup sesame seeds

1 teaspoon organic sugar

1 teaspoon kosher salt

Gomasio, a traditional Japanese condiment made from roasted sesame seeds crushed with salt, was embraced by the health food scene in earlier decades—so many East Village health-food restaurants in New York City would feature a glass shake top with the stuff *instead* of table salt. But it's so much more than a salt substitute! I've updated this blend with toasted almonds and a touch of organic sugar for a habit-forming sweet, salty, toasty, nutty dust to rain on nearly anything, especially, of course, salad.

In a small skillet over medium heat, toast the blanched almonds. Stir constantly until the almonds are a light golden brown and pour into a large mortar bowl. Watch carefully; once the almonds begin to turn golden, they will darken rapidly.

Add the sesame seeds to the skillet and roast for about 2 minutes, or until lightly roasted. The seeds will burn even faster than the almonds, so don't snooze on this! Add the toasted sesame to the almonds and add the sugar and salt.

Use the pestle to pound the mixture together, crumbling the almonds into a rough powder. Cool the mixture completely and pour into a jar with an airtight lid. For maximum freshness, store in the fridge and use within a week.

variation

Try this with black sesame, or half white and half black sesame.

Substitute hemp hearts for the almonds for a nut-free version.

the
SALADS

GREEN, CRISPY, CRUNCHY, CHEWY

The seasonal-themed salads that kick off this chapter are for those times you crave "a nice big salad." Piles of leafy, fluffy, crisp, and crunchy greens—you got it. Yet greens are just the beginning (essential, sure, but a part nonetheless); greens are the canvas for bold dressings; filling, protein-rich toppings; crunchy toasted bread; and substantial roasted or marinated veggies and fruits. Pile it on! Use this chapter as inspiration to build the salad bar of your dreams, a scoop of this and a drizzle of that for forkful after forkful of flavor-popping goodness.

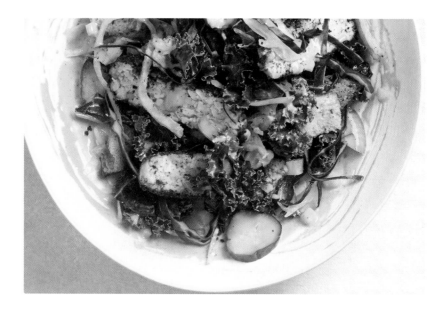

THE BRIGHT AND SPICY SPRING ASPARAGUS SALAD

Serves 3 to 4

CHOOSE A DRESSING

Hemp Seed Caesar Dressing (page 31)

Ginger Garlic Fire Dressing (page 57)

Wasabi Miso Lime Dressing (page 56)

Tahini French Dressing (page 45)

The Best Orange Balsamic Vinaigrette (page 72)

TRY ONE OR MORE OF THESE TOPPINGS

Tahini Miso tofu (page 92) or Peruvian Chile Lime tofu (page 87), sliced into batons

Salt-and-Pepper Fried White Beans (page 102)

1 cup Caesar Walnuts (page 123)

SALAD

1 pound asparagus spears

2 tablespoons white wine vinegar or sherry vinegar

1 tablespoon olive oil

Generous pinch of kosher salt and freshly ground black pepper

High-heat oil for grilling

½ pound snap peas

¼ pound spring radishes (such as French Breakfast) or Japanese salad turnips, scrubbed well

4 cups arugula, spinach, or a mix of both

2 cups dandelion or chard leaves, torn or sliced into bite-sized pieces

Bitter spring greens that overwhelm CSA produce boxes are the foundation for those "return-to-life" kinds of salads much needed at the end of winter. Gild it with other spring veggies; asparagus, radishes (French Breakfast in the spring especially), and thinly sliced snap peas—you can practically eat the last chill of winter away. Even where post-holiday diets are a distant memory and gym routines stop feeling so routine after March, there's something about a big bowl of cool crunchy greens that feels exactly like the kind of springtime health kick you want to dive into headfirst.

Prepare and chill the dressing first. If using the tofu, prepare and keep chilled, or if making the beans, prepare the beans, wrap in a heatproof container, and store in the oven at 200°F to keep warm for up to 45 minutes, or until ready to serve.

When you're ready to grill the asparagus, wash and pat the spears dry. Trim about 1 inch off the bottom of each stem, if the stems are very tough and thick. Whisk together the vinegar, oil, salt, and pepper and rub the asparagus with this marinade. Reserve any remaining marinade.

Preheat cast-iron grill pan over medium-high heat (or if you own an outdoor grill, follow manufacturer's directions for setting it up). Use a silicone brush to generously brush the pan with oil as needed. Grill the

Continued

asparagus for about 2 to 3 minutes, rotating the spears occasionally; the goal is to get some nice grill marks on the spears. Gently transfer the finished asparagus onto a plate to cool.

Slice the snap peas on a bias and fluff slightly to separate the pieces. Slice the radishes as thinly as possible, or use a Japanese mandoline to slice into paper-thin pieces.

In a mixing bowl, toss together the arugula, dandelion, any remaining grilling marinade, and 2 tablespoons of dressing. Pile the salad in a large serving platter or in individual bowls. Arrange the grilled asparagus on top of the salad. Scatter over the salad the tofu or beans and, if using, a handful of walnuts. Drizzle with the remaining dressing and serve.

variation

SPRINGTIME OPTION

Fiddleheads, those tender baby fern stalks, are a beautiful seasonal garnish on this salad and can be prepared just like asparagus. Gently wash ½ pound of fresh fiddleheads and pat dry. Rub with the same marinade used for the asparagus and cook on a cast-iron pan as directed for asparagus. Fiddleheads take only a minute or so to cook and ready when bright green and tender-crisp to the bite.

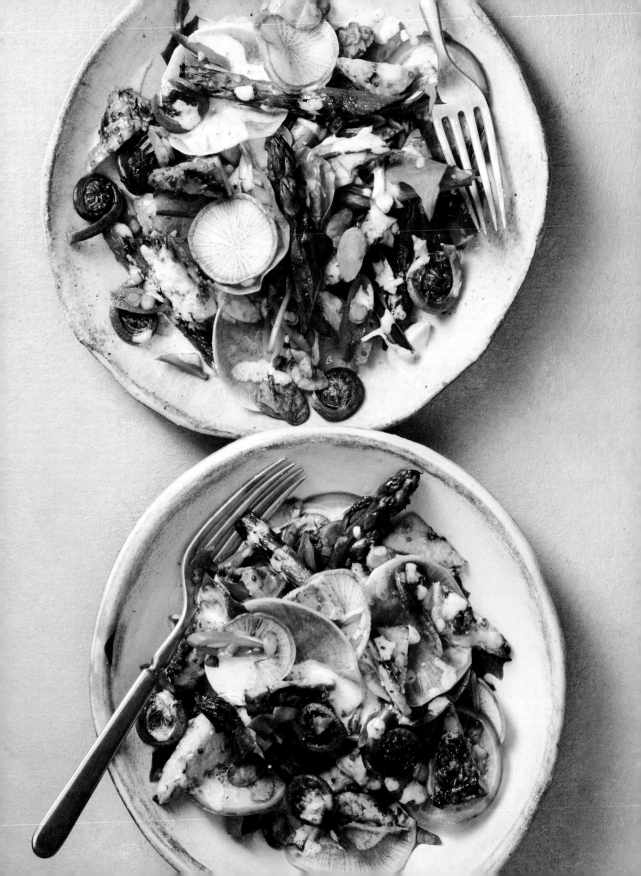

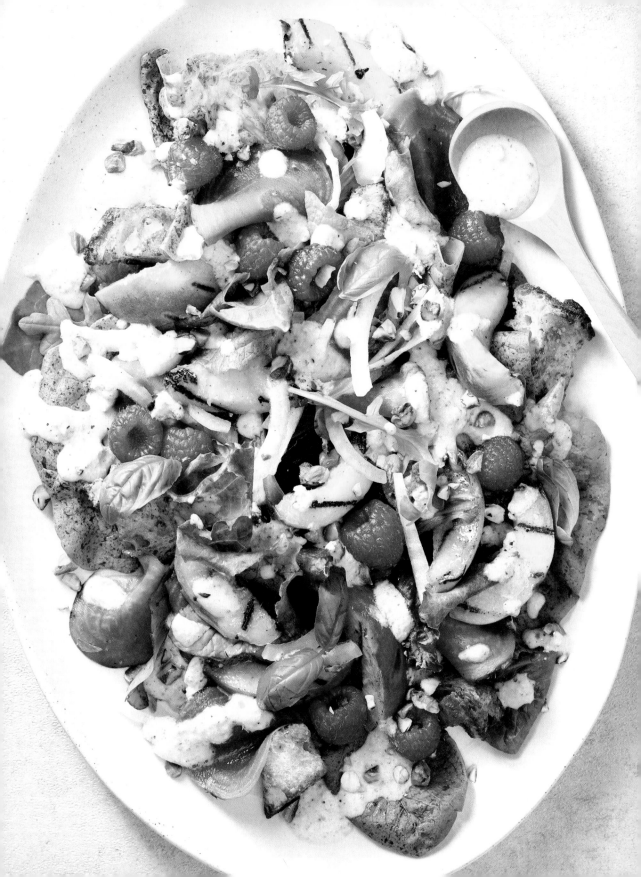

THE JUICY GRILLED SUMMER DAYS PEACH SALAD

Serves 3 to 4

CHOOSE A DRESSING

Bright and Tangy Lemon Maple Vinaigrette (page 68)

Oil-Free Cashew Lemon Pepper Dressing (page 46)

Oregano Garlic Lemon Vinaigrette (page 69)

Sriracha Cilantro Ranch Dressing (page 40)

TRY ONE OR MORE OF THESE TOPPINGS

1 cup Crumbly, Salty Almond Cheese (page 113)

1 cup Beet Prosciutto strips (page 131)

SALAD

2 pounds peaches, apricots, or similar seasonal stone fruit, ripe but still relatively firm (no mushy peaches, please)

3 tablespoons olive oil

1 tablespoon white wine vinegar

1 tablespoon lemon juice

Generous pinch of kosher salt and freshly ground black pepper

High-heat oil for grilling

4 cups romaine, butter, or Boston lettuce, washed and spun dry and torn into bite-sized pieces

2 cups arugula, washed and spun dry

1 cup basil leaves, torn and divided

1 sweet white onion, quartered and cut into ¼-inch slices

½ cup shelled green pistachios, lightly toasted and roughly chopped

½ cup ripe raspberries (optional)

There's that all-too-brief time in the summer when peaches—lots and lots of them—seem to overtake every market stand and there's little time to bake more peach pies. This is also the same time when fresh basil is in full riot mode. So into this salad they both go. Treat the peaches to a light grilling in a cast-iron grill pan (or an outdoor grill, if you are so lucky to have one) and scatter the salad with toasted pistachios and a creamy dressing. For a really spectacular dish, top with crumbles of salted almond cheese and strips of homemade beet prosciutto.

Prepare the dressing and, if using, Crumbly, Salty Almond Cheese and Beet Prosciutto in advance. Keep these chilled until it's time to serve the salad.

When you're ready to grill the peaches, wash and pat the fruit dry. Slice each peach into quarters and discard the stems and pits. Whisk together the oil, vinegar, lemon juice, salt, and pepper and rub or brush all the peach sections with the marinade. Reserve any remaining marinade.

Preheat cast-iron grill pan over medium-high heat. Use a silicone brush to generously brush the pan with oil as needed. Grill the peaches for about 2 minutes on each side, turning only once; the goal is to get some nice grill marks on each side but not cook so much that the peach completely falls apart. Use a metal spatula to gently transfer finished slices onto a plate to cool. If the peaches are rather large (4 inches or wider), slice quarters into thinner, bite-sized slices.

Continued

When the peaches are all set, in a mixing bowl, toss together the lettuce, arugula, ½ cup basil leaves, onion slices, any remaining grilling marinade and 2 tablespoons of dressing. If desired, roll up the slices of the beet prosciutto; for smaller pieces, overlap a few to create more-or-less same-sized rolls. Pile the salad in a large serving platter or in individual bowls. Arrange the grilled peaches with the beet prosciutto (if using) on top of the salad. Scatter over the salad the almond cheese (if using that too) along with the remaining basil leaves, toasted pistachios, and ripe raspberries, if using. Drizzle with the remaining dressing and serve this beauty right up!

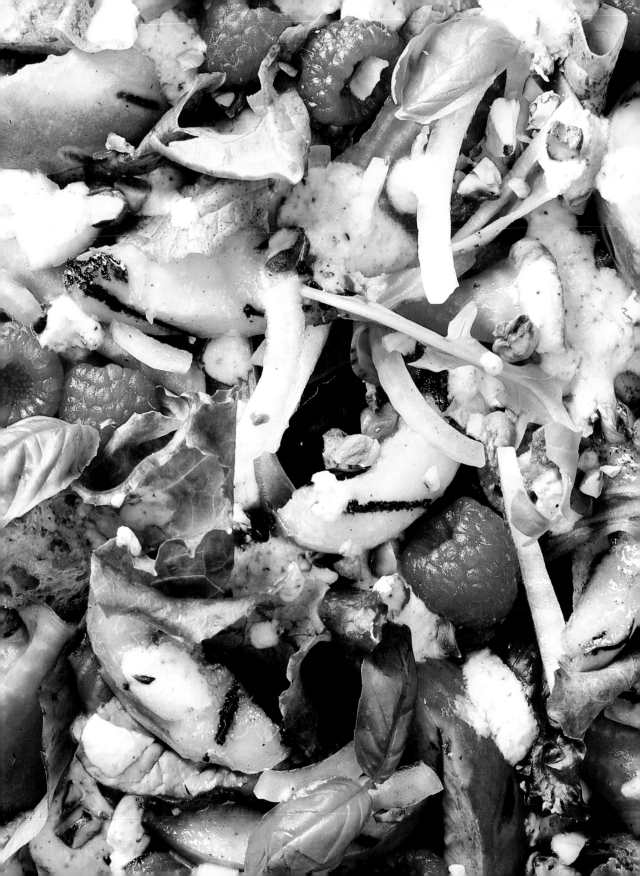

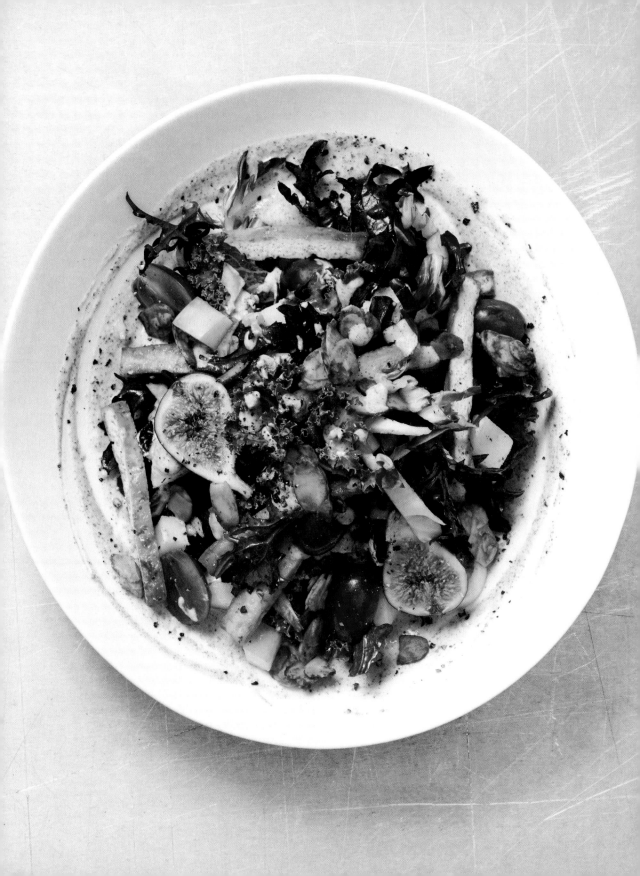

THE BIG CRUNCHY AUTUMN VIBES SALAD

Serves 3 to 4

CHOOSE A DRESSING

Oil-Free Cashew Lemon Pepper Dressing (page 46)

The Best Orange Balsamic Vinaigrette (page 72)

Maple Mustard Shallot Vinaigrette (page 70)

Red Pepper and Almond Romesco Dressing (page 52)

TRY ONE OR MORE OF THESE TOPPINGS

6 slices Golden Coriander Bird tofu (page 93), sliced into batons

1 cup Crispy, Cheesy Almond Crunch (page 117) or 1 cup toasted pecans

2 cups Herbed Cornbread Crunch (page 145) or Simple Croutons (page 140)

SALAD

6 cups mix of romaine lettuce and curly kale, cleaned and torn into bite-sized pieces

2 cups thinly sliced radicchio

1 cup diced ripe pear or red or green apple, unpeeled

1 cup thinly sliced celery

½ cup dried cranberries or 1 cup red grapes, sliced in half

4 fresh figs, sliced in half

This fluffy salad is layered with all the rustic flavors of fall: apples, Cheddar-flavored crunchy nuts, kale, toasty cornbread croutons, and a touch of sweetness from red grapes or dried cranberries.

Batons of mellow and aromatic Golden Coriander Bird tofu and a zesty, creamy drizzle of a citrus dressing, a roasted red pepper Romesco dressing, or a robust mustard dressing top this full entrée salad. Packed with sweet and savory flavors and bountiful textures, it's so easy for this salad to become a year-round favorite.

Prepare the dressing and tofu, almonds or pecans, and croutons in advance. Keep these chilled (except the croutons, which will be fine on the counter) until it's time to serve the salad.

When it's time for the salad, in a large mixing bowl, combine the croutons, lettuce and kale mix, radicchio, pear or apple, celery, and cranberries or grapes with 2 tablespoons of dressing. Use tongs to vigorously toss together to combine. Portion out the salad into large serving bowls. Arrange the tofu batons over each portion, scatter the nuts over the tofu, and garnish with the figs. Drizzle with any remaining dressing and serve pronto!

THE BOLD AND BOUNTIFUL WINTER SALAD

Serves 3 to 4

CHOOSE A DRESSING

Hollyhock Dressing (page 61)

New Catalina Dressing (page 62)

Tahini French Dressing (page 45)

Hemp Seed Tarragon Dijon Dressing (page 32)

TRY ONE OR BOTH OF THESE TOPPINGS

Maple Almost Like Bacon tempeh or tofu, sliced into batons, or seitan, diced (page 94)

Root Bacon (page 127)

SALAD

1 large red or blue potato, sliced thin or diced

1 tablespoon extra-virgin olive oil

Pinch kosher salt

2 cups Salad Rice (page 105)

1½ cups diced, unpeeled ripe pear or tart eating apple

2 cups diced fennel

2 cups shredded lacinato (dinosaur) kale

4 cups thinly shredded red, green, or savoy cabbage

1 cup Bacon Crunch pecans (page 121) or just plain toasted pumpkin seeds

Chunky winter vegetables, crunchy apples, and chewy rice get crispy, cool, and fresh with lashings of flavorful, richly textured dressing and smoky bacon flavors. Tempeh was the overall favorite protein served with this salad, but pick your favorite! Proof yet again that salads can be hardworkin' lumberjack food. Or just-cozy-in-your-flannels-on-the-couch-and-watch-the-snow-fall-and-pretend-you're-a-lumberjack food.

Prepare and chill the dressing first. If using the tofu, prepare and keep chilled. If using the root bacon, prepare in advance and keep chilled. If desired, re-crisp the bacon briefly by either heating it in a dry cast-iron skillet over medium heat for about 2 minutes, flipping once, or warming it in the oven at 325°F for 5 to 7 minutes.

Preheat oven to 400°F and on a small baking sheet toss sliced potato with olive oil. Spread in a single layer, sprinkle with salt, and roast, flipping once, for 12 to 14 minutes until golden. Prepare the rice close to serving time.

When it's time for the salad, in a large mixing bowl, combine rice, pear or apple, fennel, kale, roasted potato, and cabbage with 3 to 4 tablespoons of dressing. Vigorously toss together to combine. Portion out the salad into large serving bowls. Arrange the tofu batons over each portion, and scatter the pumpkin seeds and the root bacon over the tofu. Drizzle with any remaining dressing, button up your flannels, and dig right in.

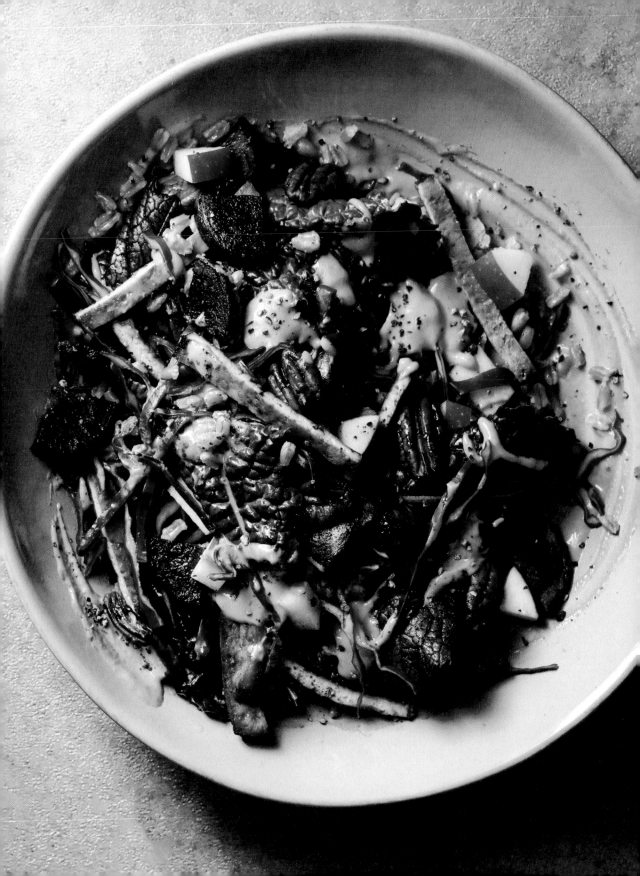

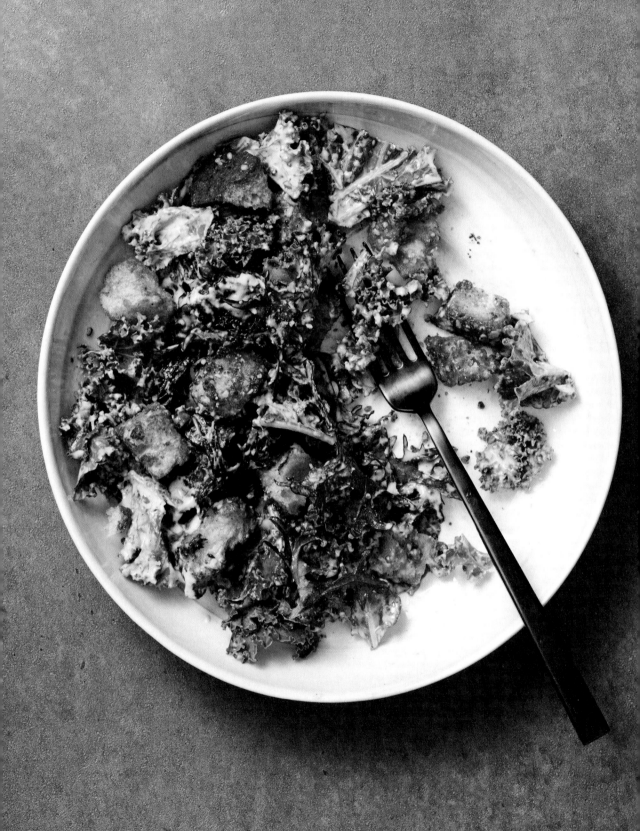

FOREVER KALE CAESAR WITH CHEESY, CRISPY CROUTONS

Serves 2 to 3

3 cups Cheesy,
Crispy Croutons
(page 142)

Toasted Sun and
Pepita Parm
(page 110)

Hemp Seed Caesar
Dressing (page 31)

1½ pounds curly
kale

Somewhere in the last ten years, kale salad—namely, kale Caesar—became the darling of the entire salad-eating universe. And with so many versions having crossed, mingled, and crossed again and again, we can be certain that kale Caesar salad will be savored forever, or until the last salad spinner on earth winds its final rotation.

I've made many versions of vegan Caesar salads over the years, but this one is richer and fattier and tangier and bolder. Perfect with just the kale or as a bed for a highly seasoned roasted tofu or perhaps a handful of sliced red grapes, or cucumbers, or tomatoes, or whatever you can imagine goes great in, around, or on top of this hearty salad. And of course, the kale can be kicked out completely in favor of traditional crunchy romaine lettuce.

Make the Cheesy, Crispy Croutons first. They can be prepared up to a month in advance (croutons have a long life until you start eating them by the handful), so why not just make them well in advance? You can also prepare the Toasted Sun and Pepita Parm a week ahead too. See? Halfway done, and you're already a week ahead on the schedule for this salad.

When it's time to make the salad, prepare the Hemp Seed Caesar Dressing, and chill it until you're ready to dress the greens.

Continued

Tear the leaves off the kale, then wash and spin the leaves dry. Tear the kale into bite-sized pieces. Transfer the kale to a big mixing bowl and spoon on 3 tablespoons of the dressing. With tongs or your fingers, massage the dressing into the kale for about 1 minute. Add the croutons, a few tablespoons of the parm, and the remaining dressing. Use tongs to toss the ingredients and moisten everything with the dressing.

Portion the salad into serving bowls and sprinkle on a healthy dusting of more parm before serving.

variation

CLASSIC ROMAINE CAESAR

Swap out romaine for the kale; opt for a 1-pound head of the freshest romaine lettuce you can find. Slice the lettuce into quarters and trim away the tough core. Chop each quarter into hearty 2-inch ribbons or tear into bite-sized pieces. Wash, spin dry, and proceed as directed for salad.

RESTAURANT-STYLE ENTRÉE CAESAR

Just before serving, top with any flavor of baked tofu, tempeh, or seitan, sliced into thin strips. Just like in a restaurant (well, only a vegan one), but without the upcharge for the extra protein. My favorites for this are Sriracha Orange (page 90), Golden Coriander Bird (page 93), Tahini Miso (page 92), Lemon Dijon (page 89), and, of course, Hot Sauce Buffalo (page 84).

SRIRACHA RANCH SALAD PARTY

Serves 4

CHOOSE A DRESSING

Sriracha Cilantro Ranch Dressing (page 40)

Horseradish Hemp Dressing (page 34) or New Catalina Dressing (page 62)

TOPPINGS

6 slices Maple Almost Like Bacon tofu (page 94), diced

3 cups Seedy Garlic Bread Croutons (page 139)

½ cup Bacon Crunch pumpkin seeds (page 120)

SALAD

1 large head butter or Boston lettuce, washed, spun dry, torn into bite-sized pieces

1 head iceberg lettuce, core removed and chopped

1 hothouse (English or Persian) cucumber, peeled, seeded, and thinly sliced

1 pint cherry tomatoes, cut in half

1 red onion, peeled and sliced into paper-thin half-moons

3 to 6 pickled pepperoncini peppers (Italian pickled peppers), cut into ¼-inch slices

½ cup minced chives

This salad? It's a salad that doesn't take itself too seriously and knows what fun is. It's a big chopped salad, a stadium rock concert of a salad of crisp iceberg lettuce, cucumbers, tomatoes, croutons, bacon-flavored veggies, and the kicker: a spicy, creamy sriracha-infused dressing with chewy nuggets of "bacon"-flavored tofu. It's the ideal salad for piling into burrito-sized tortillas for wraps (make sure to grill the tortilla to soften it up before rolling) or serving on a plain vegan-cheese pizza. *Did she just say on the pizza?* See my variation below!

Prepare the dressing at least an hour in advance and chill well until ready to use. Prepare the baked tofu, pumpkin seeds, and croutons in advance. Keep the tofu chilled, and keep the croutons and the seeds at room temperature until it's time to serve the salad.

When it's time for salad, in a large mixing bowl, combine both lettuces, the cucumber, tomatoes, onion, and pepperoncini with 3 to 4 tablespoons of dressing. Vigorously toss together to combine. Portion out the salad into large serving bowls or spread on a large round platter.

Arrange on top of the salad the diced tofu, croutons, and pumpkin seeds. Drizzle with the remaining dressing and sprinkle the minced chives, and let the salad party commence!

Continued

variation

SALAD PIZZA

There's an unusual pizza slice that still roams some old-school slice shops of New York City. Salad pizza is exactly what it sounds like . . . a plain cheese slice with a topping of simple salad: tomato, iceberg lettuce, a slice of onion, and a pickled Italian pepper, usually dressed with a dash of olive oil, red wine vinegar, and oregano.

While sriracha and bacon-like flavors are not typical of salad pizza, this salad channels those slice shop vibes. If you're feeling adventurous, why not try arranging a bit of this salad on top of your next homemade (or baked from frozen; sometimes it's like that) plain vegan-cheese pizza?

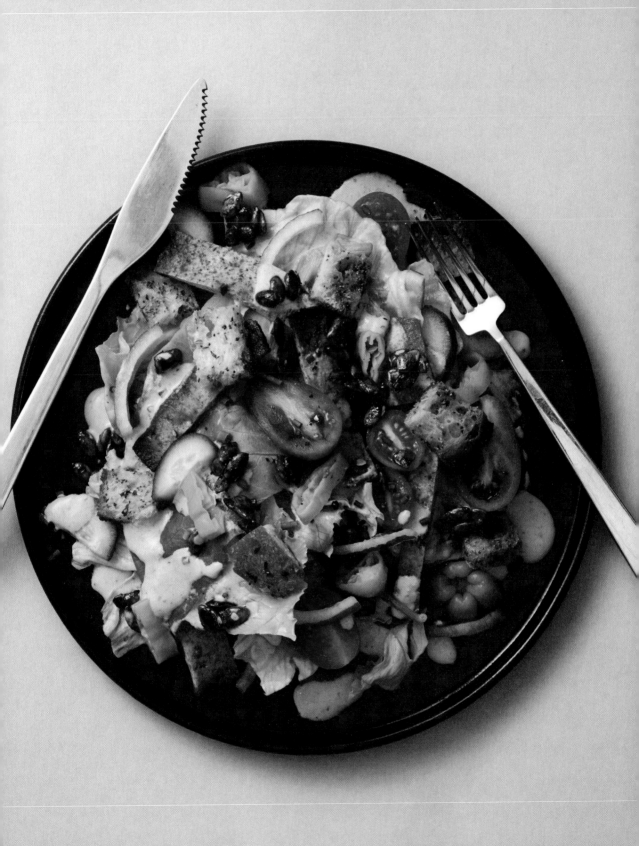

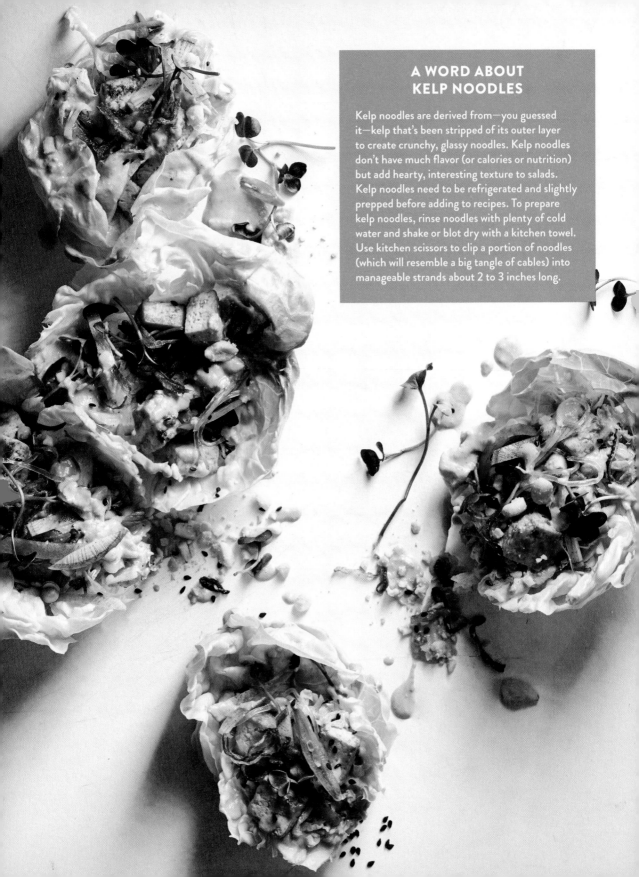

A WORD ABOUT KELP NOODLES

Kelp noodles are derived from—you guessed it—kelp that's been stripped of its outer layer to create crunchy, glassy noodles. Kelp noodles don't have much flavor (or calories or nutrition) but add hearty, interesting texture to salads. Kelp noodles need to be refrigerated and slightly prepped before adding to recipes. To prepare kelp noodles, rinse noodles with plenty of cold water and shake or blot dry with a kitchen towel. Use kitchen scissors to clip a portion of noodles (which will resemble a big tangle of cables) into manageable strands about 2 to 3 inches long.

SRIRACHA TOFU LETTUCE WRAPS WITH PEANUT DRESSING

Serves 4

TOPPINGS

6 to 8 slices Sriracha Orange tofu (page 90) or Korean BBQ tofu (page 86)

Sultry Peanut Coconut Dressing (page 54)

1 cup Crispy Lime-and-Salt Shallots (page 135)

SALAD

2 teaspoons high-heat cooking oil, such as safflower or sunflower

2 cups napa cabbage, sliced very thin

1 cup snow peas, sliced very thin on a bias

1 cup prepared kelp noodles (see note)

½ cup paper-thin slices watermelon radish, daikon, or Japanese turnips

2 scallions, ends trimmed and sliced paper thin

1 tablespoon lime juice

2 teaspoons tamari

½ teaspoon toasted sesame oil

½ teaspoon kosher salt

½ cup roughly chopped cilantro

2 tablespoons black sesame seeds

8 to 10 large lettuce leaves, such as butter, Boston, or large iceberg lettuce leaves

½ cup microgreens

Part salad, part stir-fry, and always fun to eat, lettuce wraps are the original handheld salad. A fabulous use for our misunderstood but loyal friend iceberg lettuce, butter, and even small collard leaves work just as well to cradle a scoop of crunchy seared cabbage slaw interwoven with spicy tofu, crunchy fried shallots, and an irresistible peanut sauce. One of the recipe testers said it best with, "My husband requests this weekly."

Dice the tofu into ¼-inch cubes, prepare the dressing, and keep both chilled until ready to serve. The dressing will thicken up after more than an hour in the fridge; if desired, loosen it up a little by whisking in a tablespoon of warm water before serving.

Heat a wok over high heat and add the oil. Add the cabbage and stir-fry just long enough to gently wilt the cabbage and sear some of the tips. Immediately dump the cabbage into a large mixing bowl and add the snow peas, kelp noodles, sliced radish or turnip, and scallions. In a small bowl, whisk together the lime juice, tamari, sesame oil, and salt. Pour over vegetables and add the cilantro and the diced tofu. Toss the salad again and heap into a large serving dish. Sprinkle the top of the salad with sesame seeds, fried shallots, and microgreens.

Serve with the peanut sauce on the side and the lettuce leaves stacked on a separate plate. To eat, grab a leaf, scoop on the salad, dollop on a healthy scoop of the peanut sauce, fold, and stuff it in your mouth!

CHICKPEA PICKLE COLLARD WRAPS

Makes 4 wraps

DRESSING

Hemp Seed Caesar Dressing (page 31)

SALAD

2 (15-ounce) cans chickpeas, drained and rinsed

1 red, tart apple, core removed and finely diced (do not peel)

1 cup celery, thinly sliced

1 cup minced dill pickle, plus 1 to 2 teaspoons pickle juice

½ cup fresh dill or flat-leaf parsley, roughly chopped

½ cup minced red onion or sweet white onion

1 teaspoon celery seed

Fresh cracked pepper and kosher salt as desired

4 large collard leaves or 2 heaping cups of baby spinach leaves

4 soft lavash-style whole-wheat bread wraps or burrito-sized whole-wheat tortillas

Never was much of a tuna salad fan, but chickpea salad prepared almost like tuna salad has won the hearts of vegans, chickpea fans everywhere, and me.

Minimalist in mayo content but packed with bright veggies, herbs, and, brilliantly, pickles, wrapped in collards (or engineered as a melt on toast), is still one of my favorite brown-bag lunches. The collards provide a moisture-resistant barrier between the moist salad and the wrap, plus it adds a delightful layer of green crunch. No collards? Large spinach leaves stand in beautifully.

Prepare the dressing; the dressing can be used immediately in this recipe or made up to 3 days in advance and chilled until ready to use.

In a large mixing bowl, mash the chickpeas just enough to break up the beans. I prefer a chunky texture with a few random whole beans, but chop as fine or chunky as desired. Add the prepared dressing, apple, celery, pickle, dill or parsley, onion, and celery seed. Add a few generous twists of black pepper and use a rubber spatula to mix well. Taste and adjust the seasoning of the salad with a little extra pepper, a dash of salt, or a drizzle of the reserved pickle juice, if desired.

Assemble each wrap. Lay out the wraps and, if using collard leaves, lay the leaves flat and slice away the tough stems (the easiest way is to fold the leaf in half along the stem and slice off). If necessary, trim each leaf to the same length of the wrap and lay the leaf on top of the wrap.

Continued

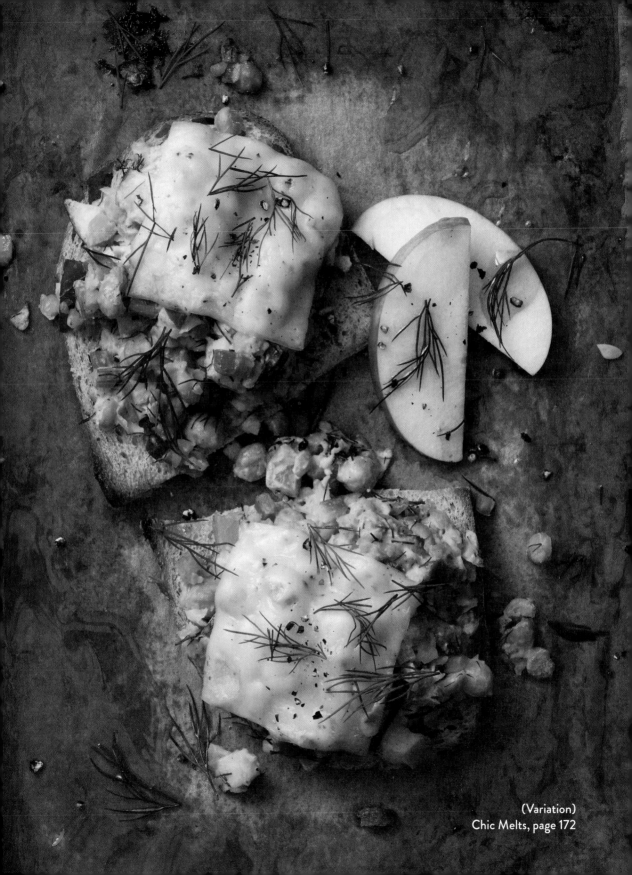

(Variation)
Chic Melts, page 172

Scoop about a cup of the salad onto the bottom third of the collard or wrap and roll up like a burrito: Fold the lengthwise outer edges inward about an inch, then use your fingers to firmly tuck the roll inward and roll into a nice plump tube. If you're bringing it to work or on a day hike, wrap it tightly in foil and chill until you're ready to rock!

variation

THE CHICKPEA OF THE SEA

Long for some ocean flavor in your wrap? Add half a sheet of toasted nori seaweed (sushi wrap seaweed) to your wraps. For another boost of maritime flavor, add 1 teaspoon of toasted dulse seaweed powder along with the spices into the chickpea salad.

CHIC MELTS

Cool chickpea salad loves to snuggle under a blanket of melted vegan cheese in this open-face sandwich. Scoop the salad onto toasted marble rye slabs and top with a slice or two of your favorite melty vegan cheese. Broil under high heat for 2 minutes, or until the cheese bubbles and browns.

ORANGE COLLARD GREENS, CORN, AND BLACK-EYED PEAS

Makes 3 to 4 large servings

DRESSING

The Best Orange Balsamic Vinaigrette (page 72)

TOPPINGS

3 to 5 tablespoons of crumbled Crumbly, Salty Almond Cheese (page 113)

Marinated or baked tempeh (page 77) made with Peruvian Chile Lime (page 87) or Sriracha Orange (page 90)

1 cup Herbed Cornbread Crunch (page 145)

Pan-Roasted Chile Corn (page 134)

SALAD

2 cups black-eyed peas, drained and rinsed

14 ounces to 1 pound thinly shredded collard greens

½ cup thinly sliced red or yellow onion

½ cup dried cranberries

Freshly cracked black pepper, to taste

Sweeter than kale and loaded with calcium, assertive collard greens deserve some salad appreciation too. Just like kale or your average stressed-out city dweller, collards mellow out after a massage (a tangy orange dressing massage for collards, that is). The dressing works out any lingering anxieties in this beneficial green; salty, tender crumbles of Crumbly, Salty Almond Cheese and roasted corn pamper tenderized collards, which in turn take care of you.

Prepare the crumbled almond cheese and chill the dressing until ready to serve. Make the tempeh and cover to keep warm until ready to serve. Or you can cook and chill the tempeh a day in advance and gently warm it once again on the stove top before you're ready to serve.

In a large mixing bowl, toss the black-eyed peas with half of the dressing. Set aside to marinate for about 20 minutes. Add the shredded collards, onion, and dried cranberries to the bowl. Toss with the dressing, and use your fingers to lightly massage the collards with the dressing until the greens are tenderized.

To serve, mound in each serving plate about half a serving of the greens. Sprinkle with some of the almond cheese, half of the roasted corn, and a few cubes or triangles of the tempeh, and drizzle on a little dressing.

Continued

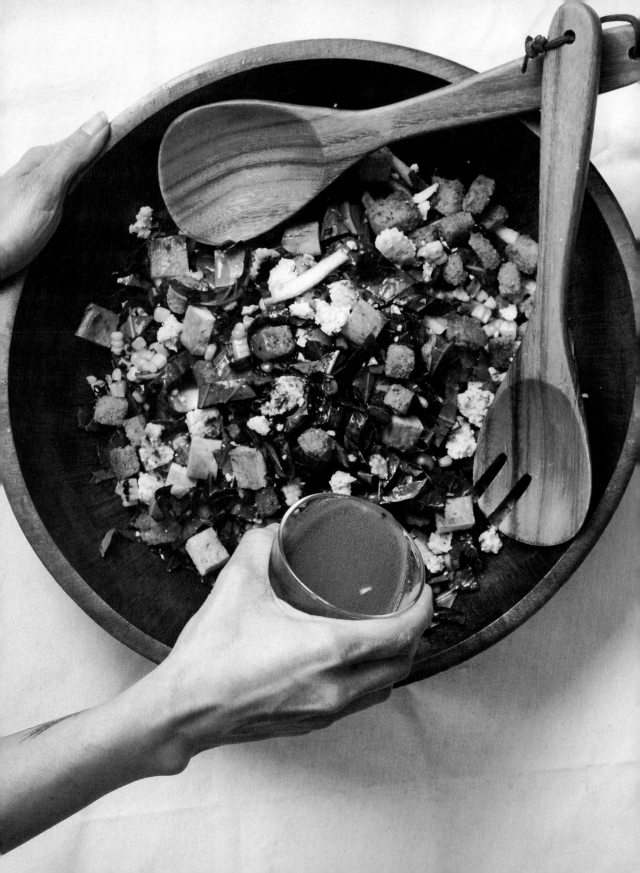

Top with more collards (for a full serving), then arrange a few more cubes or triangles of the tempeh, the remaining corn, and a few more crumbles of the almond cheese. Dust each serving with a little freshly cracked pepper and serve, passing around the remaining dressing.

BUFFALO TOFU, BUTTERNUT SQUASH, AND KALE BOWL

Serves 2 to 3

CHOOSE A DRESSING

New Catalina Dressing (page 62)

Tahini French Dressing (page 45)

Bright and Tangy Lemon Maple Vinaigrette (page 68)

TOPPINGS

6 to 8 slices of Hot Sauce Buffalo tofu (page 84)

1 cup Bacon Crunch hazelnuts (page 121)

SALAD

1 to 1½ pounds butternut squash, peeled and seeds discarded

1 tablespoon olive oil

½ teaspoon pumpkin pie spice

½ teaspoon sea salt

A few twists of cracked pepper to taste

4 cups kale, torn into bite-sized pieces

2 cups shredded red cabbage

1 red onion, quartered and cut into ¼-inch slices

The combination of roasted butternut squash and chewy hot sauce tofu is easy to love and will win over eaters of any persuasion (vegan or otherwise). A step up from the usual kale salad and dressed with sweet and smoky glazed hazelnuts, this salad tastes like fall but is worth revisiting all year long.

Prepare the Hot Sauce Buffalo tofu and keep warm. Preheat the oven to 400°F. Dice the squash into ½-inch-wide chunks. On a large baking sheet (or two smaller sheets, the ingredients divided between each sheet), mound the squash and drizzle with the oil, pumpkin pie spice, salt, and pepper. Toss to coat the squash chunks with the oil and spices, then spread into a single layer. Roast for 20 to 25 minutes, stirring occasionally, until squash is meltingly tender and browned on the edges. Remove from the oven to cool slightly. It's also possible to roast the tofu while you bake the squash, as they both cook at the same temperature. Give yourself an extra 15 minutes to get both done before serving time.

While the squash is roasting, prepare the dressing. Place the kale, cabbage, and onion in a large mixing bowl. Dice the tofu into ¼-inch pieces and add to the bowl.

While the squash is still warm, add to the mixing bowl along with half of the dressing. Use long-handled tongs to thoroughly coat the salad with dressing. Divide among serving bowls and sprinkle with chopped nuts.

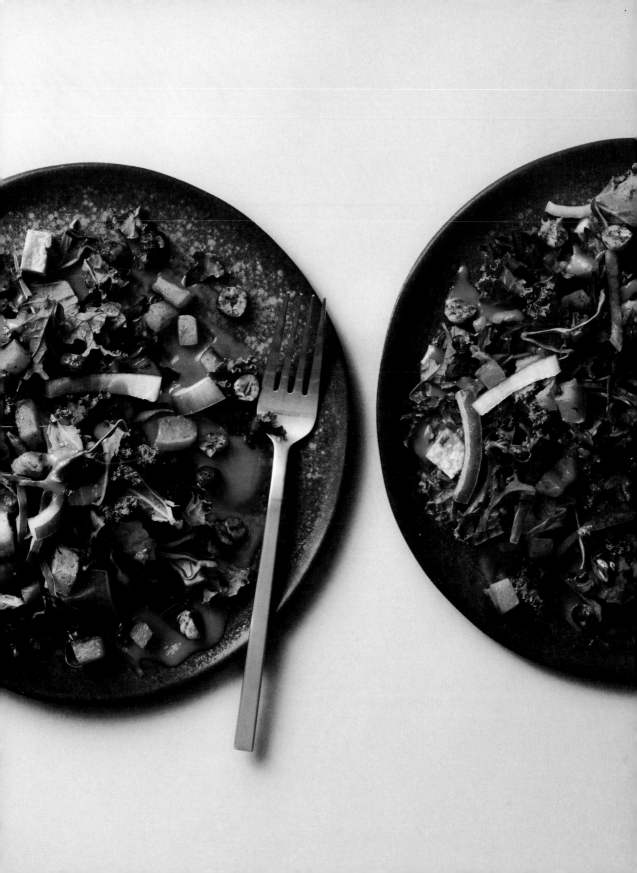

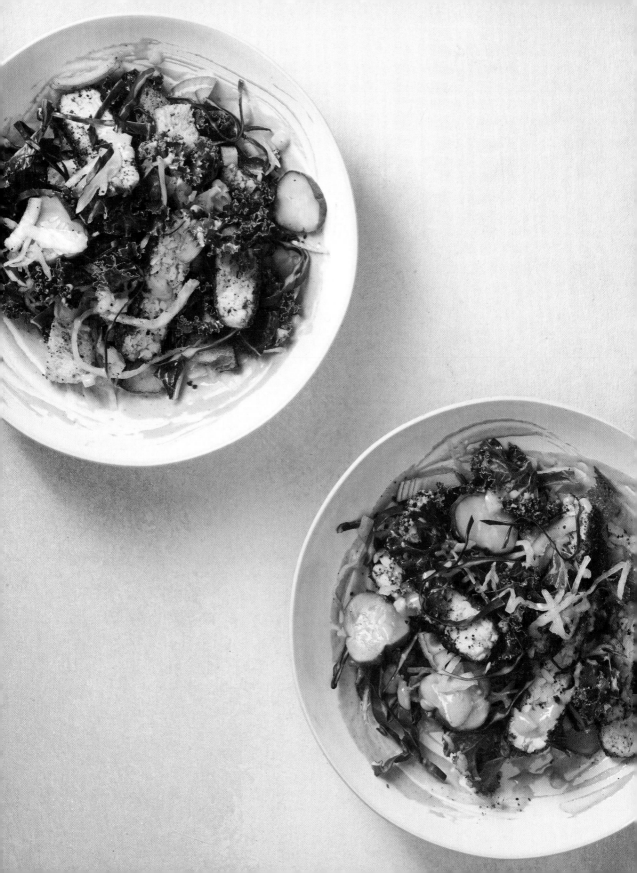

BLACKENED TEMPEH REUBEN SALAD

Serves 2 to 3

CHOOSE A DRESSING

Horseradish Hemp Dressing (page 34)

Tahini French Dressing (page 45)

TOPPINGS

Whole-Loaf Blackened Tempeh Pastrami (page 97), sliced very thin

Any style of crouton, preferably made with marble rye bread

SALAD

6 cups ruffled kale, washed, spun dry, torn into bite-sized pieces

2 cups thinly sliced red cabbage

1 sweet white onion, quartered and thinly sliced

1 kosher or half-sour pickle, thinly sliced

The tempeh Reuben salad in my first book created a fire in me to perfect the whole deconstructed-sandwich-as-a-salad experience. Compelled to give it another spin, this revised salad is intensified with a blackened pastrami-style tempeh and a spicier, less sweet Russian (or velvety Tahini French) dressing. If you feel like garnishing the top of each salad bowl with a little mound of sauerkraut, that would be an inspired decision, but the salad sits up straight with a heaping of diced deli pickles and sliced white onions.

Prepare the dressing and chill until ready to dress the greens. Keep the prepared vegetables chilled until ready to serve. Prepare the blackened tempeh and slice into thin strips.

In a large bowl, toss the kale, cabbage, and onion with half of the dressing. Pile into large serving bowls. Garnish the top of the bowl with fans of the sliced tempeh, and garnish with pickles and croutons. Serve right away and pass around the remaining dressing.

ROASTED, GRILLED, AND HEARTY SALADS

S alads should never be limited to just raw vegetables. Roasting, grilling, and occasionally frying salad toppings is essential for memorable entrée salads. Sizzling hearty proteins contrast with cool, crunchy veggies and create unforgettable and highly craveable main dish entrées. Elevate that average plate of lettuce and tomatoes to a zesty bowl of anticipation!

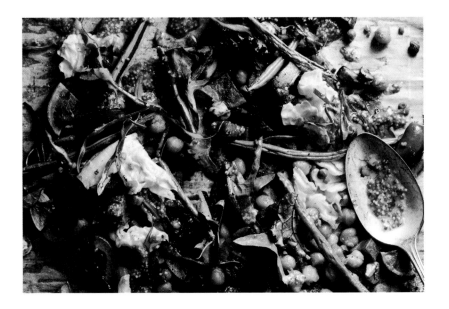

THAI BASIL SPAGHETTI SQUASH WITH CURRY TOFU

Serves 2 to 3, depending on your feelings about spaghetti squash

DRESSING

2 garlic cloves, peeled

½ teaspoon kosher salt

1 to 2 Thai bird chiles, fresh or dried

1 shallot, peeled and chopped

1-inch cube of peeled ginger

2 tablespoons coconut sugar

2 tablespoons tamari

¼ cup freshly squeezed lime juice

CHOOSE A TOPPING

Sweet Lime Curry tofu (page 91) or Sriracha Orange tempeh (page 90)

SALAD

2 to 2½ pounds spaghetti squash

2 cups mung bean sprouts or shredded napa cabbage

1 hothouse (English or Persian) cucumber, peeled, sliced in half, seeds removed, and sliced into thin half-moons

1 cup julienned carrot

2 scallions, thinly sliced

1 cup coarsely chopped cilantro, divided

½ cup coarsely chopped mint, divided

½ cup coarsely chopped Thai basil (or any fresh basil), divided

1 cup roasted, chopped unsalted cashews

Lime wedges, for garnish

Spaghetti squash: Never has a humble vegetable been loaded with so many expectations. Is it *just like* pasta? I don't think so. But once oven-steamed, those tender yet assertive noodle-like squash strands are great when splashed with the sought-after Thai flavors of lime, soy sauce, cilantro, and spicy Thai basil—and garnished with succulent curry lime tofu. No Thai basil? Then any fresh basil is fine. Spaghetti squash understands.

In a mortar and pestle, mash together the garlic, salt, chiles, shallot, ginger, and coconut sugar into a chunky paste. Drizzle in the tamari, then work in the lime juice a tablespoon at a time. Taste the dressing, and if needed, spark it up with a splash more of tamari or drizzle of lime juice.

Wash the outside of the squash, pat dry, and slice in half (a cleaver is great for attacking this hard squash). Preheat the oven to 400°F, and find a glass or ceramic baking dish that can nest the two squash halves. Arrange them cut-side down into the dish and pour about 1 inch of water into the dish; the combo of baking with a water bath will steam-roast the squash, ideal for crisp-tender strands. Slide into the oven and roast for about 35 to 40 minutes, or until a sharp knife can easily pierce the squash. To check the doneness of the squash strands, flip over a half and use a fork to pluck out some strands. The strands should be al dente, tender but firm.

Continued

Remove from the oven and flip over the halves. When they are cool enough to touch, use a fork to gently scrape out the strands and transfer them to a mixing bowl. Add the sprouts, cucumber, carrot, scallions, and half of the cilantro, mint, and basil. Pour on the dressing, and use long-handled tongs to fold the salad ingredients into the dressing.

Shape mounds of the squash salad onto serving platters; try "twirling" the strands with the tongs for more attractive mounds with added height. Arrange the slices of tempeh or tofu alongside the squash. Scatter the cashews and the remaining fresh herbs on each serving. Present with lime wedges and an open mind about the probability of pasta from a vegetable.

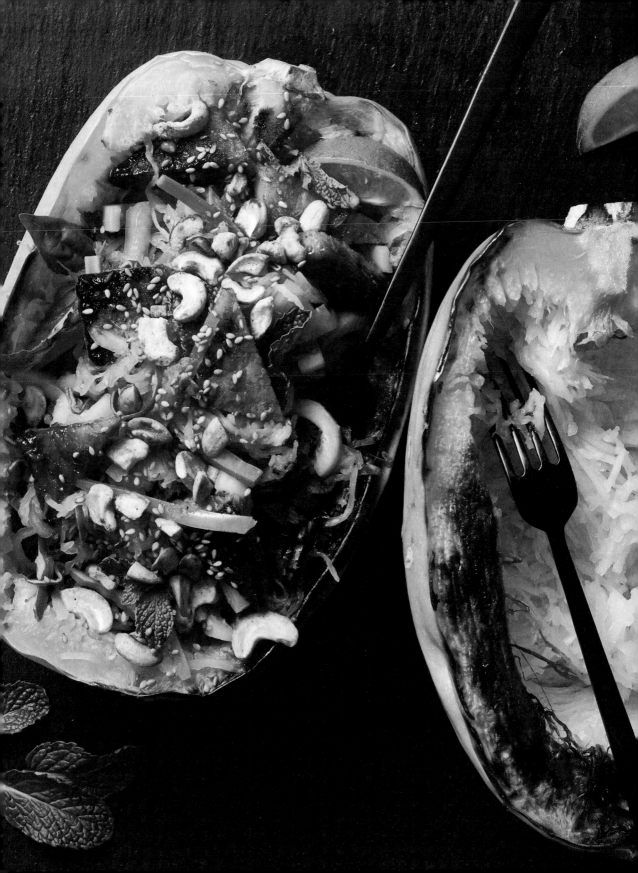

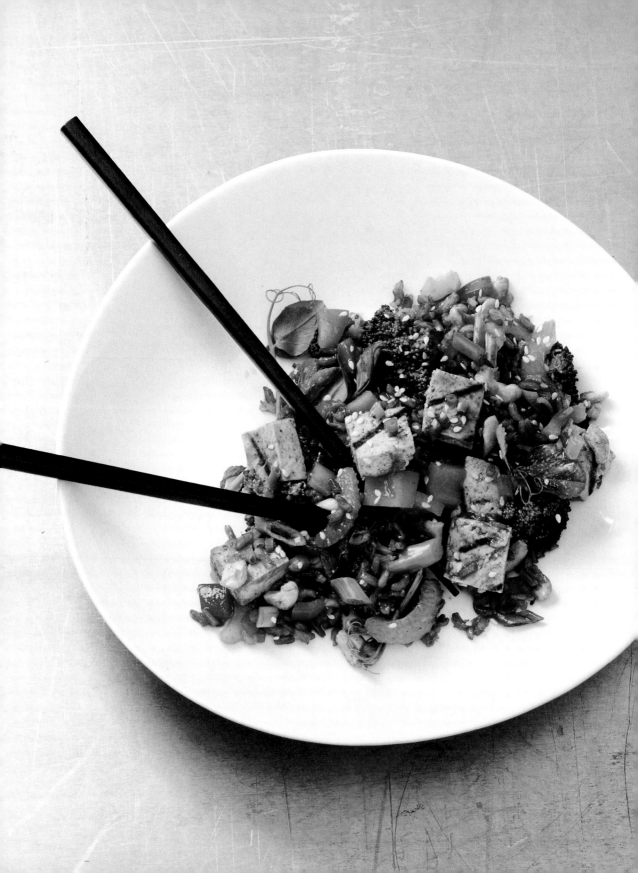

GENERAL TSO'S TOFU AND BROCCOLI SALAD

Serves 2

DRESSING

Deep Dark Sesame Dressing (page 55)

TOPPINGS

6 to 8 slices of Sriracha Orange (page 90) or Savory Sesame Tamari (page 85) tofu

SALAD

1 tablespoon kosher salt

4 cups broccoli florets, cut into bite-sized pieces

1 red bell pepper, seeds removed and sliced into matchsticks

2 stalks celery, sliced thin on a bias

2 scallions, white and tender green parts, sliced thin on a bias and divided

1 cup pea shoots, roughly torn (optional)

1 recipe Salad Rice (page 105) made with short-grain brown rice

1 cup 7-Spice Peanuts (page 111)

Salad inspired by classic American-Chinese restaurant fare has become something of an obsession. The American-Chinese classic General Tso's (Insert Favorite Vegan Protein) is my default when ordering Chinese takeout. It's also the inspiration for this salad centered around emerald-green gently blanched broccoli, chewy brown rice, baked tofu, and sweet and garlicky hoisin sauce dressing. The spicy vinegar-laced peanuts add a boom of fatty crunch. Do you always ask for 4-red-chile-pepper-level heat when ordering General Tso? Whisk in 2 or more tablespoons of sriracha into the Deep Dark Sesame Dressing!

Bring a 2-quart pot of water to boil over high heat, and fill another large bowl with cold water and keep it close by. Add the salt to the boiling water, then add half of the broccoli florets and blanch for about 30 seconds; the broccoli will turn bright green. Use metal tongs or a spider skimmer to immediately transfer the broccoli to the bowl of cold water; this stops the cooking process by cooling down the broccoli. Repeat with the remaining broccoli. Drain the broccoli into a colander and vigorously shake the colander to remove excess water, or blot the broccoli dry with a clean kitchen towel.

Cut the tofu slices into ¼-inch cubes and transfer to a large mixing bowl. Add the broccoli, bell pepper, celery, half of the scallions, pea shoots, if using, and cooled rice, and drizzle with half of the dressing. Toss to coat with dressing.

Divide salad among serving bowls. Drizzle on the remaining dressing, then garnish with a lavish helping of the peanuts and the remaining scallions. Serve at room temperature.

ROASTED CABBAGE STEAK WITH PEANUT SAUCE AND FRIED SHALLOTS

Serves 2 to 3

DRESSING

Sultry Peanut Coconut Dressing (page 54)

MAKE THE TOFU AND PICK A TOPPING

2 cups finely diced Savory Sesame Tamari (page 85) or Korean BBQ (page 86) tofu, tempeh, or seitan or Maple Mushroom Bacon (page 125)

Crispy Lime-and-Salt Shallots (page 135)

Coconut Turmeric Lime chips (page 138)

SALAD

1½ pounds (1 big head about 7 inches in diameter) savoy or green cabbage

2 garlic cloves, peeled

2 teaspoons

kosher salt

⅓ cup freshly squeezed lemon juice

2 tablespoons mild olive oil

A few twists of ground black pepper

1 pound hothouse (English or Persian) cucumbers, diced

½ pound red radishes, diced

1 jalapeño pepper, seeded and sliced into matchsticks

2 scallions, thinly sliced

1 cup cilantro, lightly packed and roughly chopped

1 package soba noodles, cooked until al dente, rinsed and chilled until ready to serve (optional)

Teetering between vegetable steak and salad, these slabs of roasted crinkly savoy cabbage drenched in smooth peanut coconut dressing and crunchy fried shallots are beautiful topped with a marinated cucumber and radish salad. Bits of diced tamari tofu or—even better—shiitake bacon make it filling. Alternatively, it's great served on a bed of lightly dressed soba noodles for a heartier dish. Serve these beauties with a steak knife and fork, or chop the cabbage sections into bite-sized pieces for maximum chopstick grab potential.

Prepare the dressing and your toppings (tofu, shallots, and/or coconut chips) of choice; keep chilled until ready to use. Trim away the dried-out, tough stem of the cabbage, but leave the core intact. Slice the cabbage into sections about 2 inches wide. Preheat the oven to 400°F and line baking sheet(s) with foil. Place cabbage slices on the foil about 2 inches between each section; this will help them roast and brown nicely—too close together and the cabbage will steam (instead of roast) and become soft and pale, rather lightly browned and crisped on the edges.

In a mortar and pestle, mash together the garlic and salt. Transfer the paste to a small mixing bowl and whisk in the lemon juice, oil, and black pepper. Drizzle half of the mixture on the cabbage steaks, flipping over and coating the other sides. Rub the dressing into the crinkles of the cabbage. In a large mixing bowl, combine the cucumber, radish, jalapeño, and scallions and toss with the reserved dressing. Cover and chill this salad until showtime!

Slide the cabbage into the preheated oven and roast for 30 minutes, flipping each section halfway through. The cabbage is ready when it is browned in patches and tender. Remove it from the oven and use a wide spatula to transfer the cabbage steaks to serving plates, about 2 or 3 per serving. Whisk the peanut sauce to loosen it up (add a tablespoon or two of hot water if needed) and drizzle about 2 tablespoons on each serving. Top with the cucumber salad, tofu, and mushroom bacon/shallots/coconut chips. Serve with the additional peanut dressing on the side.

ROASTED NIÇOISE SALAD

Makes 2 generous entrée salads

CHOOSE A DRESSING

Maple Mustard Shallot Vinaigrette (page 70)

New Catalina Dressing (page 62)

Balsamic Dijon Vinaigrette (page 71)

TOPPING

Roasted Lemon Pepper Chickpeas (page 100)

SALAD

2 tablespoons extra-virgin olive oil

1 tablespoon sherry vinegar or white wine vinegar

½ teaspoon kosher salt

A few twists of freshly ground black pepper

1 pound small (or tiny!) red, blue, or yellow waxy potatoes, thoroughly scrubbed

½ pound green beans, stems trimmed away

4 cups mixed greens, mesclun salad mix, chopped Boston or romaine lettuce, or other fluffy, tender greens

⅓ cup niçoise, Kalamata, or other nice European olive, pits removed

⅓ cup toasted sliced almonds or toasted chopped hazelnuts

2 heaping tablespoons capers

The renowned niçoise salad—potatoes, green beans, other Mediterranean veggies, and protein with a Dijon mustardy dressing—has the makings of a complete entrée, but prepping each thing individually can feel fussy. *When do I boil what now? What goes next to green beans? In which order do I eat each thing?* Roasting the main ingredients together on one sheet hopefully puts some of those pesky questions to rest, at least on a bed of tasty greens.

The essentials (potatoes, green beans, mustard dressing, olives, capers) remain, but the addition of roasted chickpeas and a sprinkle of Toasted Sun and Pepita Parm (page 110) make this salad casual yet exciting enough to savor in your dressiest yoga pants.

Preheat the oven to 400°F. Line a large baking sheet with foil or parchment paper. Whisk together the olive oil, vinegar, salt, and pepper. Dice the potatoes into 1-inch chunks and spread on the large pan (or one smaller pan), drizzle with half of the oil-and-vinegar mixture, and toss to coat. Roast the potatoes 20 minutes, remove the sheet from the oven and push the potatoes to one side of the pan, add the green beans, and drizzle and toss to coat with the remaining mixture.

Roast for 15 minutes, stirring the beans and potatoes occasionally. The green beans and potatoes are ready when they are tender and lightly browned. Remove from the oven and set aside to cool while you jump into the last steps!

In a mixing bowl, combine the salad greens with a big spoonful of Maple, Catalina, or Balsamic dressing; use long-handled tongs to dress the greens. Divide among serving plates, then pile on the potatoes, chickpeas, and green beans over the greens and casually flourish the olives, nuts, and capers on top. Drizzle on the dressing and eat!

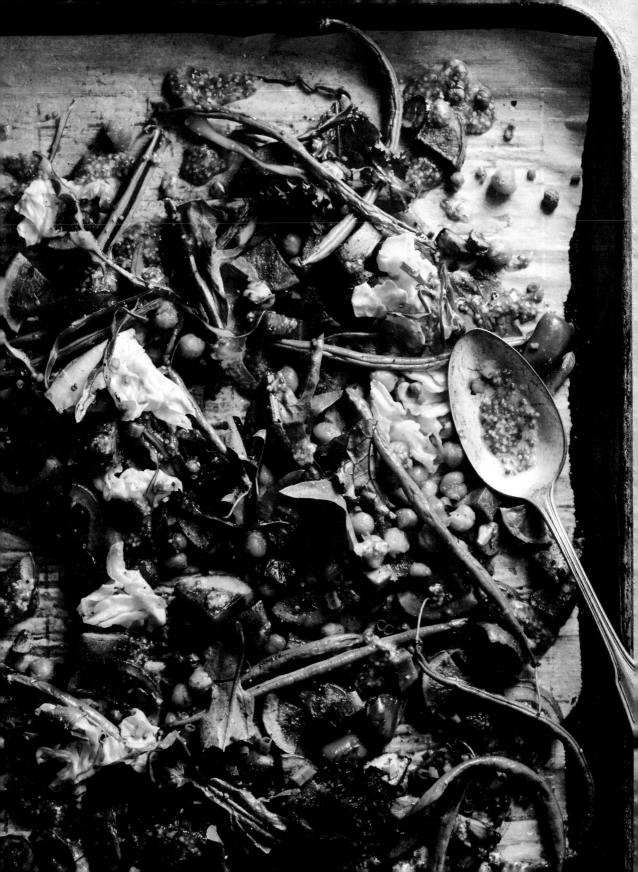

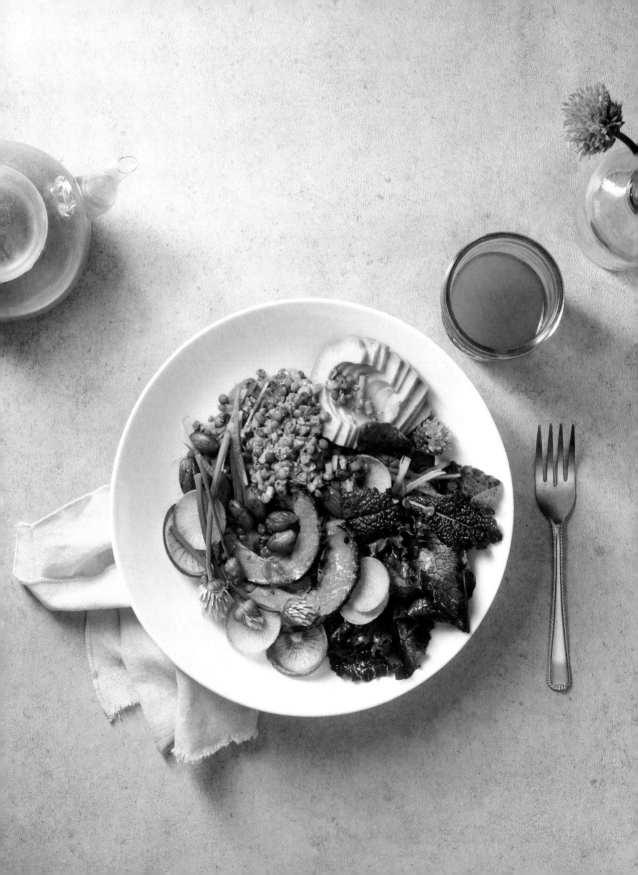

PROTEIN-PACKED SALAD FOR BREAKFAST

Makes 1 serving

CHOOSE A DRESSING

Keep It Simple Vinaigrette (page 67)

Bright and Tangy Lemon Maple Vinaigrette (page 68)

Oregano Garlic Lemon Vinaigrette (page 69)

Ginger Garlic Fire Dressing (page 57)

Tahini French Dressing (page 45)

New Catalina Dressing (page 62)

Hollyhock Dressing (page 61)

TOPPINGS

½ ounce Bacon Crunch Nuts and Seeds (page 120), Caesar Walnuts (page 123), or any plain toasted seeds or nuts

SALAD

3 ounces Dressed Lentils (page 104)

3 ounces Mighty and Flavorful Tofu, Tempeh, and Seitan (page 74), any flavor

2 ounces chopped spinach, kale, collards, mustard greens, or any mix of hearty greens

½ ounce thinly sliced sweet onion, bell pepper, radish, kohlrabi, fennel, or blanched green beans

1 ripe avocado, sliced

½ cup thinly sliced roasted winter or summer squash

1 teaspoon flaxseed, hemp seed, or olive oil

1 teaspoon apple cider vinegar

A few twists of freshly ground pepper and sea salt (or a pinch of kosher salt)

Looking to ditch the sugar-bomb pastry breakfast, or just need to change it up from the usual fruit-and-protein-powder smoothie? This simple arrangement of tofu, lentils, greens, and dressing is the anti-doughnut (sorry, doughnut-every-day friends)—a high-protein, high-fiber, full-of-good-fats, but lower-in-carbs start to their day. Or go ahead, add some healthy carbs (I do!) with a scoop of Salad Rice (page 105). This salad uses the "scale, measure, and go" method of making a salad by weight (see Salad for Nerds, page 19).

Place a single-serving salad bowl on a digital scale and tare (set to zero) the weight. Add the lentils, tofu, greens, and, if using, sliced vegetables. Remove from the scale and sprinkle with the oil and vinegar and a little salt and pepper. Toss to coat the greens and soften them up slightly. Place the bowl back on the scale and top with nuts and drizzle with dressing. Best consumed immediately or within an hour.

tip

ROASTED SQUASH

A little roasted squash adds sweetness to this morning salad. Thinly slice ¼ pound of kabocha squash or summer squash, brush both sides with olive oil, and sprinkle with a pinch of kosher salt. Preheat oven to 375°F and roast on a baking sheet, flipping once, until tender and golden, about 8 to 10 minutes. Serve warm on the breakfast salad.

ALL-DAY BREAKFAST
NACHO SALAD BOWL

Makes 2 huge bowls or 4 smaller bowls

DRESSING

Roasted Pico de Gallo Vinaigrette (page 59)

Hollyhock Dressing (page 61) (optional but very good in this recipe)

TOPPINGS

Oven-Fried Breakfast Tofu Bites (page 95)

1 cup crumbled Crumbly, Salty Almond Cheese (page 113) or your favorite feta-like vegan cheese

Red Onion Quick Pickle (page 136)

SALAD

1 pound orange sweet potatoes or Yukon Gold or red waxy potatoes, scrubbed, unpeeled, and diced into 1-inch pieces

1 small white or yellow onion, peeled and diced

1 to 2 jalapeño peppers, thinly sliced or 1 poblano pepper, seeded and diced

1 tablespoon olive oil

1 tablespoon lime juice

1 teaspoon kosher salt

2 cups baby spinach leaves, thinly sliced chard, chopped romaine lettuce, or shredded green or red cabbage

2 cups white, blue, or yellow corn tortilla chips or Toasted Wheat Tortillas (see below)

1 ripe avocado, pit removed and sliced thin

2 red ripe tomatoes, diced

Part taco salad, part tofu scramble bowl, with a lot of salad in between! Oven-roasted scrambled tofu, potatoes, cabbage slaw, avocado and tortilla chips, and two great sauces—fresh roasted pico de gallo dressing and a "cheesy" nutritional yeasty dressing—add breakfast taco vibes to this free-form taco salad. The Crumbly, Salty Almond Cheese requires some make-ahead planning, but Crispy, Cheesy Almond Crunch (page 117) can be baked while preparing the rest of the components.

Prepare the Oven-Fried Tofu Bites, Crumbly, Salty Almond Cheese (or whichever cheese-like ingredient you choose), and dressing(s) first, up to 2 days in advance. You can also roast the tofu while you make the following potatoes.

Preheat the oven to 400°F and tear off two 12-inch squares of aluminum foil. Generously rub the dull sides of the foil with olive oil. In the center of one of the foil squares, pile the potatoes, onion, and diced peppers and sprinkle with oil, lime juice, and salt, and toss with your fingers to coat in oil. Lay the oiled side of the other piece of foil on top, and crimp the edges together to create a little package. Slide the foil pouch into the oven and bake for about 20 minutes. Remove from the oven, carefully peel back some of the foil, and take a peek; if the potatoes are easily pierced with a fork, they are done! If they are still a little firm in the center, crimp the edges of the pouch again and roast for another 5 minutes. Remove from the oven and keep it wrapped until ready to serve.

Continued

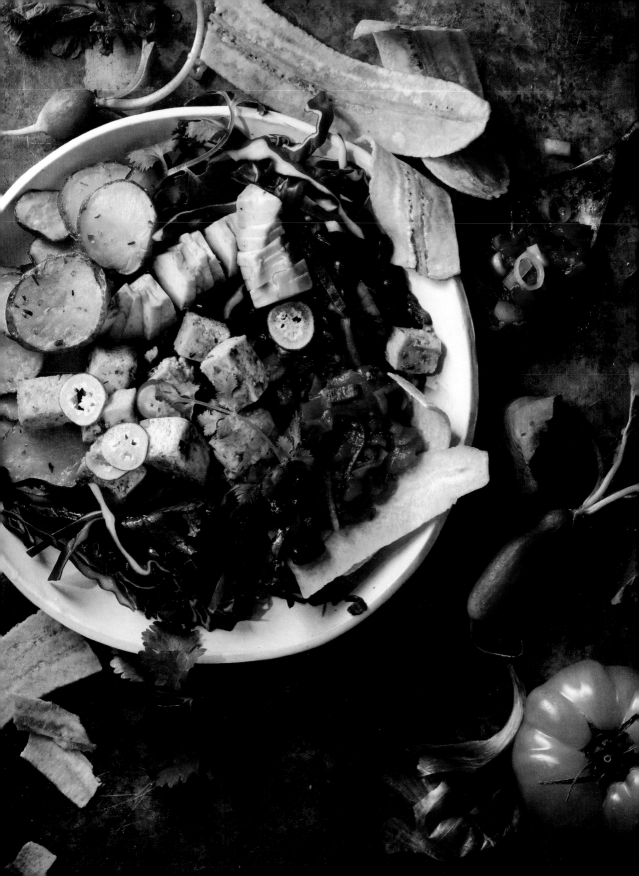

It's best to build individual servings of the salad nachos. Start each bowl with a little pile of the greens. Add a few spoonfuls of the warm roasted potatoes. Add a few tortilla chips, then a spoonful or two of the tofu cubes, then a drizzle of both dressings. Keep building the bowl up with alternating layers of salad, potato, tofu, and dressings, ending with either the potatoes or a bit of the crumble. Garnish the top with avocado slices, cheesy crumbles, pickled red onion, some diced tomato, and perhaps a sprig of cilantro. Stick a few extra tortilla chips either in the center or on the sides of the bowl for some flair. Serve right away with any remaining dressing on the side to pour on top whenever!

variation

TOASTED WHEAT TORTILLAS

Exactly what they sound like; make if you have wheat tortillas to use up and just a few minutes before serving. Simply stack the tortillas and cut into 8 triangle slices. Arrange in a single layer on baking sheets and, if desired, brush with a little olive oil. Slide into the oven just after the potatoes are done, and toast the triangles, flipping once, about 2 minutes each side until golden. Watch carefully—these can burn in the blink of an ojo!

KABOCHA AND BLACK RICE SALAD

Serves 2 to 3

DRESSING

Keep It Simple Vinaigrette (page 67), made with lime juice and rice vinegar

1 tablespoon prepared green curry paste (recipe follows)

TOPPINGS

Sriracha Orange tempeh (page 90), or Sweet Lime Curry tofu (page 91) or Savory Sesame Tamari tofu or tempeh (page 85), diced into ½-inch cubes

Sweet, Salty, Nutty Gomasio (page 148) or Coconut Turmeric Lime chips (page 138) or ½ cup roasted cashews

SALAD

1 pound peeled, cubed pumpkin or sweet winter squash

1 tablespoon mild olive oil or other neutral-tasting oil

½ teaspoon kosher salt

½ teaspoon Chinese 5-spice powder

2 cups cooked, cooled forbidden rice (see Salad Rice, page 105)

4 cups watercress (or mâche, mizuna, or tatsoi), torn into bite-sized pieces

1 cup cilantro, chopped, divided

4 scallions, white and tender green parts, thinly sliced on a bias, divided

Aromatic, earthy, and always put together in purple-black, forbidden rice is the effortless cool girl of whole grains. So I had to make sure her salad companions were worthy: sweet, savory Sriracha Orange tempeh (page 90) or Sweet Lime Curry tofu (page 91), subtly spiced roasted squash, some watercress, or maybe tatsoi or mizuna, but don't break a sweat over it. A splash of green curry vinaigrette, a shake of gomasio, a scattering of scallions. Understated and yet so stylish, cool-girl-salad status achieved, just like that.

Prepare the vinaigrette, using rice vinegar and lime juice for the choice of acids. After whisking in your oil of choice, whisk in 1 heaping tablespoon of green curry paste. Taste the dressing and adjust the seasonings with added salt, lime juice, or a touch more curry paste as needed. The dressing will be tart, spicy, and rich with herbal notes.

Preheat the oven to 400°F. Dice the squash into ½-inch cubes. Line a baking sheet with foil and mound the squash in the center. Drizzle with the oil, salt, and the 5-spice powder and stir the squash to cover with these seasonings. Roast the squash, stirring occasionally, for 30 to 35 minutes until the cubes are golden, tender, and easily pierced with a fork. Remove from the oven to cool.

In a large mixing bowl, combine the diced prepared tempeh or tofu, roasted squash, cooled rice, greens, and half of the cilantro and scallions. Drizzle half of the dressing and toss to coat. Divide into large serving bowls and garnish with the remaining cilantro and scallions and a generous amount of gomasio, coconut turmeric lime chips, or roasted cashews.

GREEN CURRY PASTE

2 teaspoons
coriander seeds

1 teaspoon cumin
seeds

1 cup firmly packed
chopped cilantro,
leaves and sprigs

1 to 2 hot green
chiles (jalapeño,
Thai, etc.)

1 shallot, chopped

2 garlic cloves,
chopped

1 tablespoon
prepared
lemongrass or
1 stalk lemongrass,
tender white part
only, chopped

1-inch piece
ginger, peeled and
chopped

½ teaspoon kosher
salt

For salad dressings, a little bit of jarred curry paste is fine, but with a bit of extra effort, a memorable and tasty green paste takes only a few minutes and uses tons of fresh, vibrant herbs.

In a small skillet over medium heat, toast the coriander and cumin seeds together until fragrant, about 1 minute. Add the seeds, along with the remaining ingredients, to a food processor and pulse into a chunky paste. Or if you're feeling like a brisk arm workout, pound into a paste in a Thai kruk (clay mortar and pestle). Use 1 to 2 tablespoons of this fresh paste in salad dressings, and freeze the rest packed in ice cube trays. Use within a month for the best flavor.

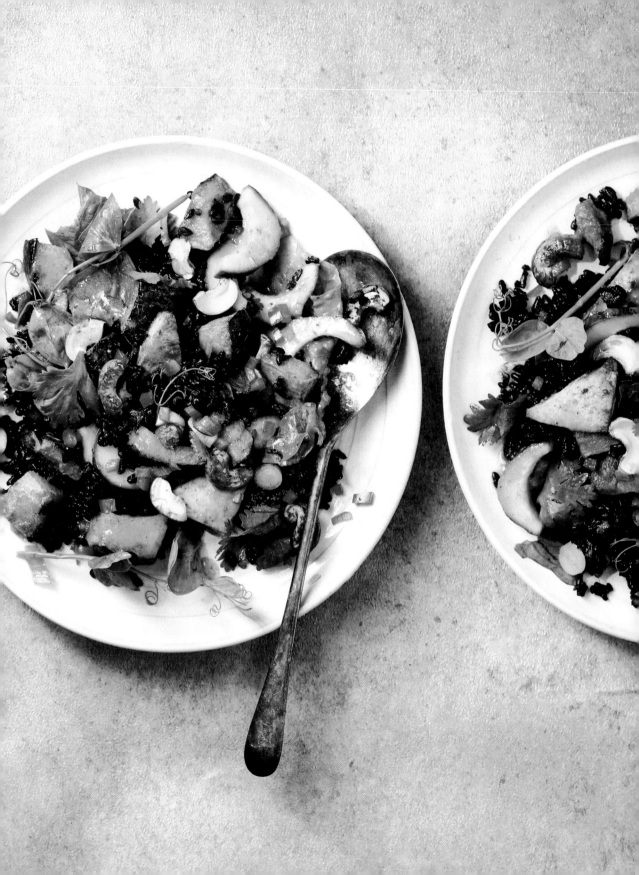

WHITE SWEET POTATO SALAD WITH SPINACH ZHUG DRESSING

Serves 2 to 3

ZHUG DRESSING

1 cup roughly chopped cilantro

½ cup roughly chopped parsley

½ cup lightly packed baby spinach leaves

1 big fat jalapeño pepper

2 garlic cloves

1 teaspoon coriander seeds

1 teaspoon cumin seeds

¼ teaspoon red pepper flakes

A few twists of ground black pepper

2 tablespoons lemon juice

1 teaspoon kosher salt

⅓ cup extra-virgin olive oil

TOPPING

1 cup Roasted Lemon Pepper Chickpeas (page 100) or diced Tahini Miso tofu (page 92)

SALAD

1 pound white sweet potatoes or Japanese sweet potatoes, unpeeled and well scrubbed

4-cup mix of 2 or more bitter leafy greens: arugula, mizuna, dandelion, watercress, or purslane, washed and spun dry

1 red onion, peeled, quartered, and cut into ¼-inch slices

With fetching wine-colored skins and creamy sweetness, white sweet potatoes are a standout improvement over their orange-fleshed siblings. Their somewhat drier texture and mellow flavor are the perfect backdrop to a bold pesto-like dressing inspired by the popular Yemeni zhug condiment, a brilliant green pesto of cilantro and fiery green chiles. This extremely hearty salad goes one step further and is piled on top of oven-roasted cauliflower steak and looks great served on a tray family-style.

Preheat the oven to 400°F and tear off a 12-inch piece of aluminum foil. Generously rub olive oil on the dull side of the foil.

Dice the potatoes into ½-inch cubes and spread in a single layer in the center of the foil. Sprinkle the potatoes with a generous dusting of kosher salt. Fold over the edges of the foil to create a little package and firmly crimp the edges. Slide the foil pouch into the oven and bake for about 15 to 20 minutes. Remove from the oven, carefully peel back some of the foil, and take a peek; if the potatoes easily pierce with a fork, they are done! If they are still firm in the center, wrap up tightly and roast for another 5 minutes. Remove the packet from the oven and partially unwrap to cool. Or for a dramatic presentation, wrap whole, unpeeled potatoes in foil and roast until tender, about 30 to 40 minutes. Keep warm until ready to serve.

Continued

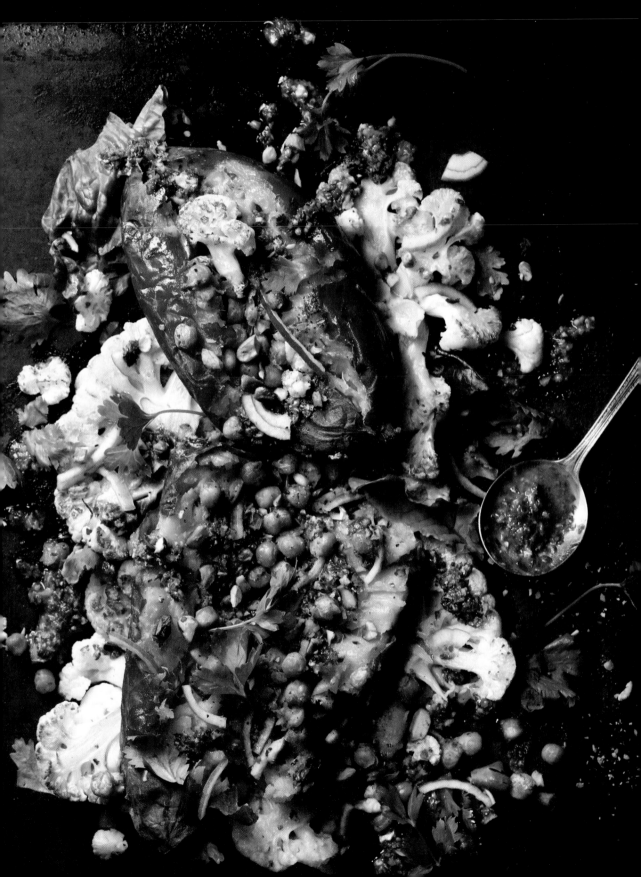

While the potatoes are roasting, prepare the zhug dressing by blending all the ingredients, except the oil, until smooth. Stream in the oil and pulse in a little at time. Chill the dressing until it's time to serve the salad.

If you're feeling ambitious and want to serve this with cauliflower steaks (and why not? The oven is on anyway!), get the steaks roasting in the oven now as well (see tip).

And when salad time arrives, spread the cleaned greens on a platter or in large individual serving bowls. Top the greens with portions of roasted sweet potatoes or, if using, slice whole potatoes in half and fill with toppings. Top with chickpeas or tofu and slivers of red onion (and cauliflower steak, if serving). Drizzle on the zhug! Serve right away and pass around the extra dressing.

CAULIFLOWER STEAKS, AN ANTI-RECIPE

Cauliflower steak is a delicious and pretty cool-looking version of roasted cauliflower. More technique than recipe, let this not-a-recipe be your guide.

Preheat the oven to 400°F and spread a sheet of foil on a baking tray. Grab a big head of cauliflower; a monster 8- to 9-inch head will make about 4 to 5 dramatically big steaks and plenty of little tidbits to nibble on. Remove the bottom leaves and ½ inch of very tough stem from the bottom. Don't, whatever you do, hollow out the core stem—this is needed to help the cauli steaks hold their shape.

Holding the cauliflower firmly on the cutting board, cut thick slices, around 1½ inches, working from one end to the other end. Crumbled florets will happen, and if your cuts are lucky today, behold, as 3 to even 5 brain-like cross sections of cauli await.

Arrange the steaks on the foil, drizzle with olive oil, patting oil into the crevices with your fingers. Flip over and rub oil on the other side. Make a little pile of the florets in a corner of the sheet, pouring on the oil too.

Generously sprinkle each steak with black pepper, smoked paprika, a bit of cumin, coriander, and a dash of garlic or onion powder. And plenty of kosher salt. Do the same to the florets pile; coat it all with goodness.

Roast for about 30 minutes, flipping halfway, until the thick center stems of the steaks are tender and juicy. Stir the florets a bit; if they get way too brown before the steak, remove them. But unless charcoal black, these bits are fantastic roasted to a deep sizzling brown. Serve steaks hot with plenty of the zhug dressing, with sweet potato salad.

ROASTED RATATOUILLE SALAD WITH ROMESCO DRESSING

Serves 3 to 4

TOPPINGS

Red Pepper and Almond Romesco Dressing (page 52)

Dressed Lentils (page 104) or Lemon Dijon baked tofu or tempeh (page 89), diced

Basil Pesto Croutons (page 140)

SALAD

1 pound eggplant

1 teaspoon kosher salt, plus more for sprinkling

3 tablespoons olive oil, divided

2 teaspoons dried oregano, divided

Freshly ground black pepper

2 red bell peppers

1 pound young zucchini

1 small bulb fennel, cut in half

1 pint cherry tomatoes, cut in half, or 2 red ripe tomatoes, diced

1 cup basil leaves, lightly packed, large leaves torn into bite-sized pieces

½ cup chopped flat-leaf parsley

4 cups baby arugula or 4 endive, chopped into 1-inch slices

If there's a reason to turn on the oven in the summer, this is it. This is the queen of summer salads, or just enhance winter produce with cheery summer flavors. Cherry tomatoes pan-roasted with eggplant and zucchini and served with a bright Romesco dressing remind me of caponata or ratatouille, but in a fork-ready salad form. It's also a portable, lunch-worthy salad; just make sure to pack the dressing separately and pour it on just before eating. Great with crusty bread or topped with Basil Pesto Croutons.

Do not peel the eggplant, but do trim the stem from the eggplant. Slice the eggplant into 1-inch-thick slices, then cut each slice into 1-inch-wide batons, then dice into ½-inch cubes. Transfer the eggplant cubes to a colander over the sink. Sprinkle with about 1 teaspoon of kosher salt and toss to coat. Set aside in the sink for at least 30 minutes (the older or seedier that eggplant is, the more you'll be happy you're salting it). In a colander, rinse the eggplant, shake away excess water, then spread the cubes on a clean kitchen towel and pat dry. At last, the eggplant is ready for action.

Preheat the oven to 400°F. Prepare two baking sheets and line with parchment paper or foil. Mound the eggplant on one of the sheets. Drizzle with 1 tablespoon of olive oil and half of the oregano and toss to combine. Spread in a single layer on the sheet and dust with salt and pepper.

Continued

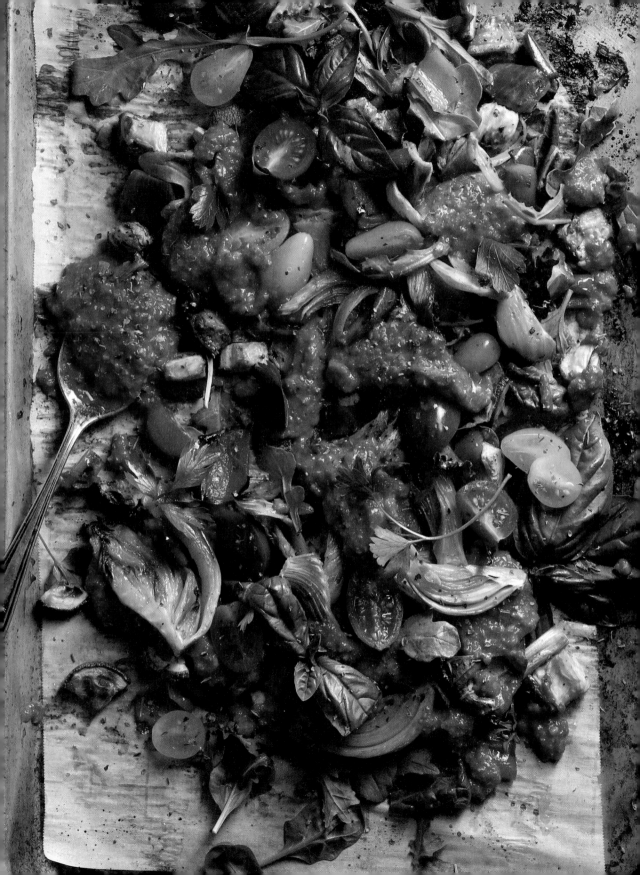

Cut the ends off the bell pepper, slice in half, and remove the seeds. Dice into ½-inch pieces. Do not peel the zucchini, just dice into ½-inch cubes. Dice the fennel halves into ½-inch pieces. Pile all these veggies onto the other baking sheet in their own piles. Drizzle the remaining oil and oregano over each veggie pile, toss veggies to coat with the oil, and spread in a single layer. Dust with salt and pepper.

Slide both baking sheets into the oven on separate racks and roast for 30 to 35 minutes, stirring occasionally. Remove each batch of roasting vegetables when they are tender and golden brown. Cool for 5 minutes, then scoop it all together into a big mixing bowl. Add the tomatoes, basil, parsley, and, if eating immediately, 2 tablespoons of the Romesco dressing. Toss to coat the veggies.

Pile the arugula or endive into a serving platter and pile on the vegetables, or create single-serving portions. Serve with the rest of the Romesco dressing and enjoy your life!

LAZY SEITAN GYRO SPINACH SALAD

Serves 2 to 3

CHOOSE A DRESSING

Cucumber Dill Dressing (page 48)

Tahini Mayo (page 43)

TOPPING

Seedy Garlic Bread Croutons (page 139), preferably made with pita strips

GYRO-FLAVORED SEITAN

8 ounces store-bought seitan or Steamed Seitan Cutlets (page 81)

⅓ cup extra-virgin olive oil

2 tablespoons red wine vinegar

2 tablespoons lemon juice

3 garlic cloves, peeled and minced

2 tablespoons tamari

1 teaspoon dried oregano

½ teaspoon ground cumin

½ teaspoon dried thyme

¼ teaspoon ground smoked paprika

1 teaspoon kosher salt

SALAD

1 head radicchio, sliced into ½-inch ribbons

4 cups baby spinach leaves, packed

1 pint cherry tomatoes, cut in half, or ½-pound red ripe summer tomatoes, cut in half and then diced

1 hothouse (English or Persian) cucumber, peeled and cut into ¼-inch slices

1 red onion, quartered and cut into ¼-inch slices

½ cup Kalamata olives, pits removed

ADDITIONAL GARNISH

Dried oregano, freshly ground black pepper, extra-virgin olive oil, 1 lemon, cut into wedges

This salad is Greek "slow" fast food; seitan (or tempeh or tofu) marinated in the essential gyro flavors of lemon-garlic-oregano, flash grilling on a cast-iron griddle, and no skewers required. Serve it with the right embellishments—creamy tzatziki-style cucumber dill sauce, olives and tomatoes, pita croutons—and nobody will care you didn't spend an extra hour poking seitan with little wooden sticks.

Make the dressing and croutons first, and keep the dressing chilled until ready to use.

Slice the seitan into ½-inch-thick strips. In a shallow baking dish, whisk together the remaining marinade ingredients. Reserve 2 tablespoons of this marinade for dressing the salad later.

Add the sliced seitan to the remaining marinade in the baking dish and flip the pieces a few times to coat in the marinade. Cover and chill for 30 minutes or overnight for maximum marinated flavor.

When you're ready to get this salad going, heat a cast-iron grill pan over medium-high heat. Use a regular cast-iron pan if a grill pan isn't available (it will be fine, just no fun grill marks). Brush the pan generously with high-heat cooking oil and layer the seitan in the pan in a single layer. Do not crowd the seitan; grill or fry for about 2 minutes until the edges are lightly browned but the seitan is still juicy, flipping and grilling each piece about 1 minute. Brush the seitan with a little extra marinade if it looks dry. Cook the rest of the strips.

In a large mixing bowl, toss the radicchio, spinach, tomatoes, cucumbers, and onion with the 2 tablespoons of the reserved gyro marinade. Arrange the salad on a platter, and arrange the gyro strips on the salad. Garnish with olives, drizzle on some Cucumber Dill Dressing, and sprinkle with plenty of oregano, pepper, and a little oil for good measure. Garnish with lemon wedges. Serve it family-style and pass around the remaining dressing (and squeeze that lemon wedge over your serving before eating) and a bowl of croutons for sprinkling.

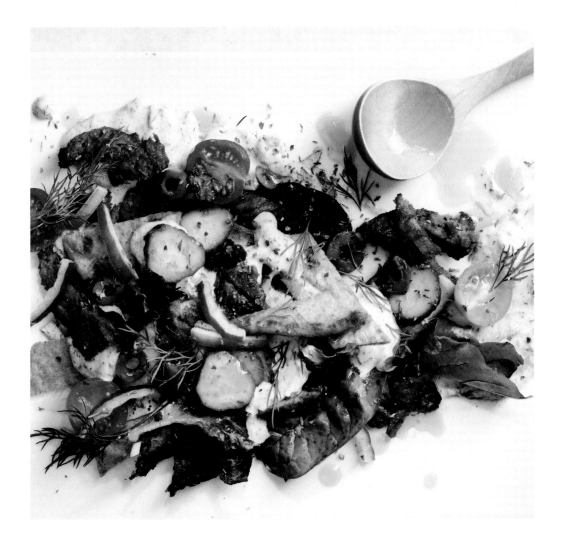

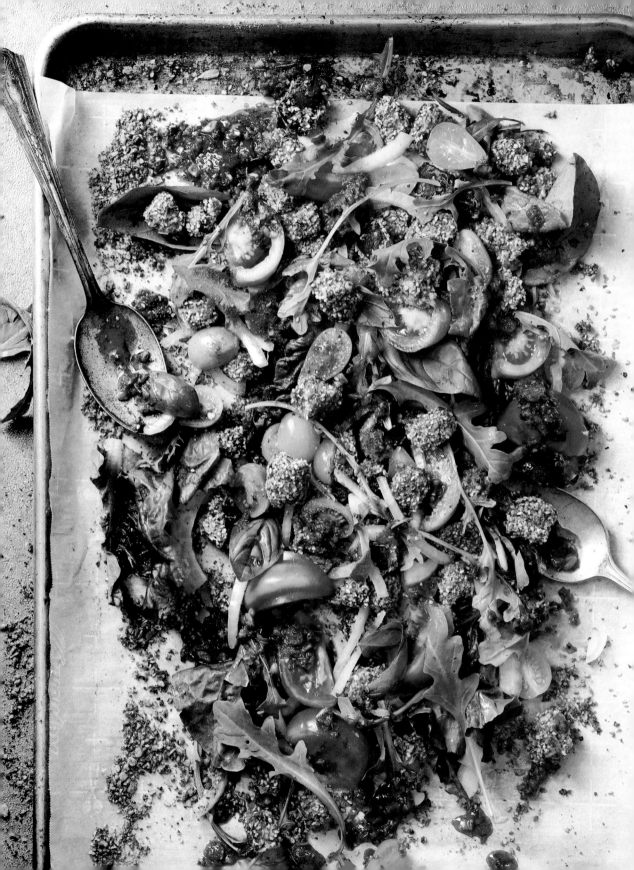

CRUNCHY EGGPLANT PARM SALAD

Serves 3 to 4

DRESSING

Sun-Dried Tomato Dressing (page 60)

TOPPING

Toasted Sun and Pepita Parm (page 110)

CRUNCHY EGGPLANT FRIES

1½ pounds Italian eggplant or 1 (8-inch) purple globe eggplant

2 teaspoons kosher salt, divided

1½ cups panko

⅓ cup nutritional yeast

1 teaspoon garlic powder

1 teaspoon dried oregano

3 tablespoons extra-virgin olive oil

⅔ cup unsweetened plain almond milk

1 tablespoon cornstarch

Olive oil cooking spray

SALAD

6 cups mix spring greens

1 head radicchio or endive, thinly sliced

1 cup cherry tomatoes, cut in half

1 cup basil leaves, lightly packed

1 small red onion, quartered and cut into ¼-inch slices

At last, a salad-based excuse to eat a big pile of extra-crunchy oven-baked eggplant cubes. A snappy sun-dried tomato dressing unites the salad things with the crisp-outside, creamy-inside cubes, so we can all agree this is still safely within salad territory. While anyone who knows a zucchini from a sneaker will never mistake this for actual eggplant Parmesan, it's incredibly tasty proof that salad can be complex, filling, and have a sense of humor.

Make the dressing and topping in advance and keep chilled.

Trim the stem from the eggplant. Slice the eggplant into 1-inch-thick slices, then dice each slice into ½-inch cubes. Transfer the diced eggplant to a colander over the sink. Sprinkle with 1 teaspoon of kosher salt, toss the cubes, and set aside to soften and drain in the sink for at least 30 minutes. In a colander, rinse the diced eggplant, shake well to remove excess water, then spread on a clean kitchen towel and pat dry the cubes.

Preheat the oven to 400°F and line a large baking sheet (or two small) with parchment paper or foil. In a large shallow dish, stir together the panko, nutritional yeast, garlic powder, oregano, and remaining salt. Drizzle the olive oil over the crumbs and massage the crumbs into the oil.

Continued

In another dish, whisk together the almond milk and cornstarch. Set up an assembly line starting with the diced eggplant, almond milk, crumbs, and lastly the baking sheets. Working with one hand and passing a few cubes of eggplant to the other, dip a few cubes in milk, then drop in the crumbs, flip a few times to coat, then drop the eggplant onto the baking sheet. Repeat with the rest of the eggplant. Do not crowd the sheets; ideally keep about ½ inch or more between cubes to help them bake crisp and golden.

Spray or drizzle eggplant generously with olive oil and bake for 25 to 30 minutes. Use a metal spatula to occasionally flip and stir the eggplant. The eggplant is done when golden and crunchy on the outside and tender in the center. Make it in batches if necessary, rather than crowd the pan with the eggplant, to prevent it from steaming and to create a crunchy exterior.

In a large mixing bowl, toss together the greens, radicchio or endive, tomatoes, basil, onion, and 2 tablespoons of dressing. In each serving dish, alternate layers of salad and eggplant cubes. Drizzle a little extra dressing on each salad, sprinkle with the Toasted Sun and Pepita Parm, and eat it while the eggplant is still warm!

PASTA AND GRAINS
WITH GREENS

Filling and luscious salads, the kind that lure in even the most salad-resistant eaters, must feature more than veggies and plant-based proteins. Yes, I'm talking about carbs. But no empty carbs here! I adore the taste and textures of bean-based pastas, whole grains and whole-grain breads, and leaving the skins on well-scrubbed potatoes and root vegetables for extra fiber, flavor, and texture. If you still think salad is wimpy, this chapter is a windfall of ideas that can bring more satisfying salads to your days and nights. And yes, even mornings.

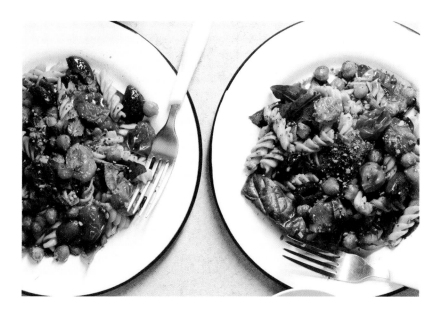

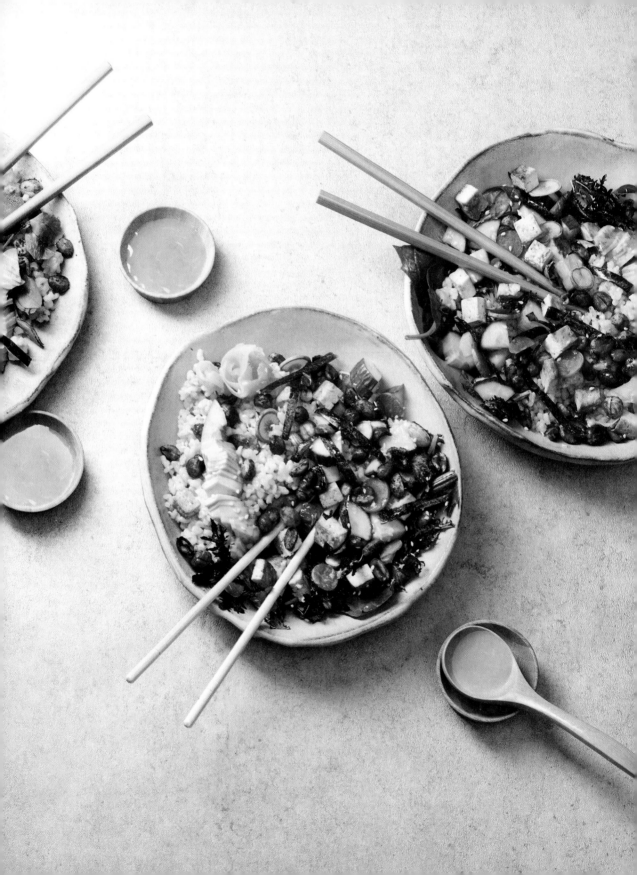

PEANUT AVOCADO BROWN RICE CRUNCH BOWL

Serves 2

DRESSING

Wasabi Miso Lime Dressing (page 56)

TOPPING

4 to 6 pieces Savory Sesame Tamari tofu or tempeh (page 85), sliced into thin strips

SALAD

2 cups cooked short-grain brown rice, warm or room temperature, or 1½ cups Salad Rice (page 105)

1 cup diced hothouse (English or Persian) cucumber

½ cup julienned or shredded carrot

½ cup roasted, preferably unsalted, peanuts or cashews, roughly chopped and divided

1 ripe Haas avocado

2 tablespoons pickled sushi ginger

2 handfuls mizuna or spring salad green mix

2 scallions, thinly sliced

1 tablespoon roasted sesame seeds

½ cup finely diced radishes or daikon

½ sheet nori seaweed, cut into matchsticks

Channeling avocado peanut rolls—the uncommon and delicious fish-free nori roll found on some creative New York City budget sushi joint menus—this comforting and flavorful whole-grain rice salad stars the satisfying duo full of good fats from avocado and protein-loaded roasted peanuts. A smooth Wasabi Miso Lime Dressing completes this bowl for nori roll lovers too lazy to roll their own.

Prepare the dressing first. In a mixing bowl, combine the warm rice, diced cucumber, carrot, and half of the roasted peanuts or cashews and drizzle on half of the dressing. Cut the avocado in half and remove the pit. Carefully peel away the skin and slice each half into very thin slices. Neatly stack the sushi ginger and slice into thin ribbons.

Divide the leafy greens into the 2 big serving bowls. Mound the rice salad into serving bowls on top of the greens. Fan out the thinly sliced avocado halves over the rice and garnish with pickled ginger, scallions, and sesame seeds, remaining peanuts or cashews, daikon/radish, and matchsticks of nori seaweed. Drizzle on the remaining dressing and eat right away!

SPICY CUCUMBER AND CURRY TOFU SALAD WITH STICKY RICE

Serves 2 to 3

TOPPING

4 to 5 pieces Sweet Lime Curry tempeh or baked tofu (page 91), sliced into thin strips

SALAD

½ cup roasted unsalted peanuts or cashews

1 pound cucumbers, preferably thin-skinned Persian or English, peeled

4 garlic cloves, peeled

2 dried Thai chiles or 2 to 3 fresh

3 tablespoons lime juice

1 tablespoon coconut sugar

1 teaspoon kosher salt

1 teaspoon white miso

6 ounces green beans or long beans, cut into 2-inch pieces (about 1½ cups cut)

½ pint cherry tomatoes, sliced in half

½ cup cilantro leaves, roughly chopped

2 tablespoons mint leaves, chopped

Steamed Sticky Rice (recipe follows)

Fresh lime juice, lots of fresh herbs, garlic, and hot chiles—the simply dressed yet endlessly versatile salads of Thailand and Laos are the greatest gift to salad lovers everywhere. This cucumber salad, garnished with a mild curry-roasted tofu, is inspired by these great Southeast Asian flavors and is a favorite weeknight dinner salad in my house. Gobs of warm sticky rice (easier homemade than you expect) are the perfect tool to mop up the garlicky cucumber salad juices.

The best version of this salad is pounded in minutes in an authentic clay Thai mortar and wooden pestle (kruk). A kruk comfortably holds 3 or more cups in the clay vessel, much bigger than a standard small marble or granite mortar and pestle. It's a fast and flexible way to make curry pastes, sauces, and even salads. Genuine kruks, while typically only available in Thai or Laotian grocery stores, are inexpensive and with a little care can last through many salads and curry pastes.

In a kruk, mortar and pestle, or food processor, pound or pulse the roasted peanuts until crumbly and transfer to a dish until ready to use.

Cut the cucumbers into 3-inch pieces, then use a mandoline with the large matchstick attachment to slice into matchstick pieces. Or use a chef's knife or julienne vegetable peeler to slice up a big pile of shredded cucumbers. It will be juicy work, so drain the juice into a glass and enjoy sips of cucumber juice while banging out the rest of this dish.

Continued

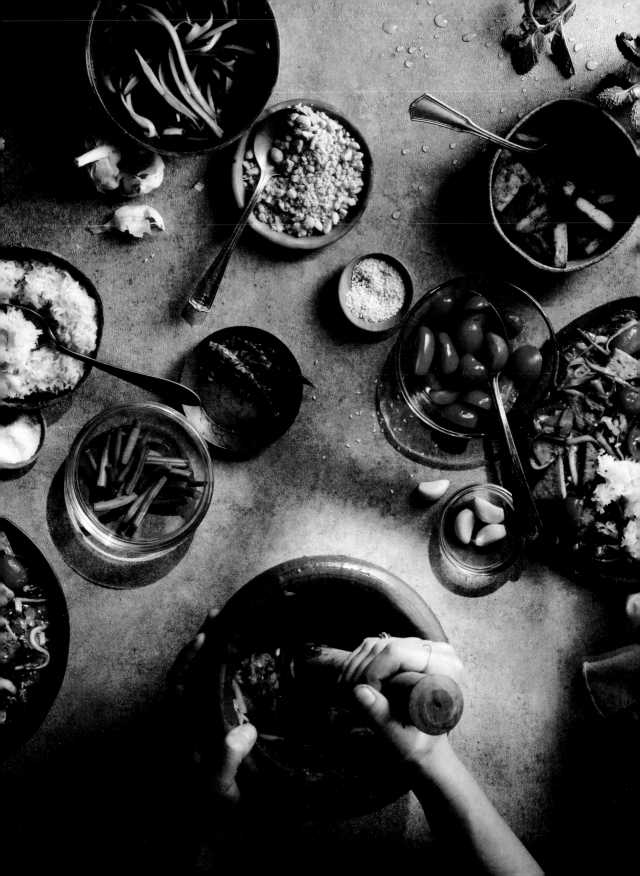

Get ready to smash things! In your Thai kruk or a big mortar and pestle (or pulse in a food processor), pound together the garlic, chiles, lime juice, coconut sugar, salt, and miso into a juicy paste.

Add the green beans and pound to flatten the beans and break them apart a little. If you're using a kruk (which is big enough to hold the entire salad), add the cucumbers and gently crush but don't go overboard; crush only enough to let the lime juice marinade work into the cucumbers. Add the tomatoes, tofu, and most of the cilantro and mint. Don't crush these ingredients; mix just enough to coat in garlic chile paste. If you are still without a kruk by now, gentle crush the green beans by rolling with a rolling pin (or pound with a can of beans) and combine in a bowl with the other ingredients.

Ladle the salad into serving bowls and garnish with a few extra leaves of cilantro and mint. Sprinkle the crushed peanuts you made forever ago over the salad servings. Serve immediately with hot sticky rice. Pinch a little ball of rice with your finger, flatten it slightly, and use it to scoop up the luscious salad and garlicky cucumber juices.

STEAMED STICKY RICE

Serves 2, about ½ cup rice per serving

1 cup sticky rice (Thai sweet rice)

Sticky rice is the easiest kind of white rice you can make. I want to holler it from a blimp circling high overhead to everyone that's ever tried to make white rice and failed. Learn this simple setup for sticky (Thai sweet) rice, and your homemade Thai dishes will thank you. Use kitchen tools you already own to rig a simple rice-steaming setup, or invest in an affordable and lovely Thai bamboo steaming basket for adventures in sticky rice for years to come.

In a mixing bowl, swish rice around with cold water a few times, draining each time, to rinse away the excess starch. Soak 1 cup uncooked sticky rice covered in 2 inches of water for 1 hour. Drain and pour the rice into a metal mesh sieve that can fit comfortably over a large saucepan. Fill the bottom of the pan with about 2 inches of water, but do not let the rice touch the water (leave about ½ inch minimum). Remove the rice sieve for now, cover, and bring the water to a rolling boil over high heat. Return the rice sieve to the pot and carefully fit it over the boiling water. Put the pot lid on top of the rice, lower the heat so that the water is now at an active simmer, and steam the rice until the grains are tender and have a semi-translucent look around the edges. Make sure the rice never touches the boiling water. If you must add more water to the pot, lift the sieve and pour in a little hot water into the pot as needed. Serve and consume the rice when it's hot, as it will toughen considerably as it cools.

Extra credit: For easier handling of the rice, and a bonus bit of flavor, line the metal sieve with a large square of banana leaf (available frozen in many ethnic markets) or bamboo leaf before adding the rice. To transfer the cooked rice, simply lift the edges of the leaf square and flip onto a serving platter, peeling and discarding the leaf when ready to eat.

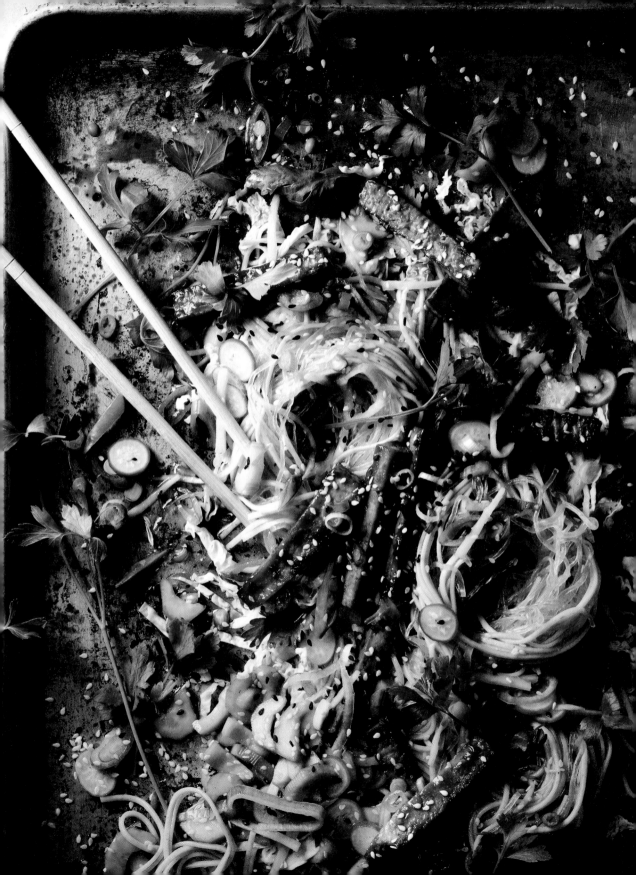

PEKING-ROASTED TOFU NOODLE SALAD

Serves 3 to 4

DRESSING

Deep Dark Sesame Dressing (page 55)

TOPPING

¼ cup hoisin sauce

1 teaspoon grated fresh ginger

Savory Sesame Tamari marinade (page 85)

1 (15- to 16-ounce) block extra-firm tofu, pressed (see page 76 for tips on pressing tofu)

NOODLES AND SALAD

6 ounces udon noodles

1 teaspoon toasted sesame oil

¼ cup rice vinegar

2 teaspoons kosher salt

2 teaspoons organic sugar

1½ teaspoons grated fresh ginger

1 pound napa cabbage

1 pound hothouse (English or Persian) cucumber

1 large carrot or 3 large radishes

4 scallions

2 tablespoons toasted sesame seeds or black sesame seeds

Inspired by Chinese takeout menus yet again, this zesty noodle salad revels in heaps of warm, roasted, glazed tofu atop juicy pickled cucumbers, scallions, and cool napa cabbage marinated in a crisp ginger–rice vinegar brine. Choose udon noodles or mix it up with crunchy kelp noodles for lighter fare. The marinade for the tofu is a hack of the Savory Sesame Tamari marinade, simply enhanced with hoisin sauce (that thick, sweet Chinese BBQ sauce available in any market store that stocks basic Asian grocery items) and a dose of fresh ginger.

Whisk the hoisin sauce and grated ginger into the Savory Sesame Tamari marinade. Drain and press the tofu for 20 minutes. Cut the pressed tofu into 12 slices.

Preheat the oven to 400°F. Pour the marinade into an 11 x 7 x 2-inch baking dish and arrange the slices in the dish (it's okay to overlap slices). Marinate the tofu slices for 5 minutes, flip them over once, and marinate for another 5 minutes while the oven preheats.

Bake the tofu for 30 to 35 minutes, flipping each slice over once at about 20 minutes. The sliced tofu is done when the marinade has been absorbed and the cutlets are rich golden brown and sizzling. Remove from the oven and cover the tofu to keep it warm. Before using the tofu in the salad, slice it into ½-inch-wide strips.

Cook the udon according to the package directions until al dente. Drain and rinse with plenty of cold water. Flip into a mixing bowl and toss with sesame oil.

Continued

In a large mixing bowl, whisk together the vinegar, sugar, salt, and grated ginger. Slice the cabbage in half, then slice each half into slender ribbons. Peel the cucumber, slice in half, scoop out the seeds with a spoon, and slice into cute ¼-inch half-moons. Scrub and julienne the carrot, or if using radishes, slice paper thin. Slice the scallions on a diagonal into thin slices. Dump the vegetables into the bowl with the vinegar marinade and use your hands to gently massage the dressing into the vegetables, especially into the cabbage. Cover and chill until ready to serve.

To serve the salad, for each portion, combine a serving of noodles with a healthy heap of marinated vegetables. Mound on serving plates and top with pieces of warm roasted tofu. Drizzle any remaining juices from the marinated vegetables over the salad and scatter over each serving sesame seeds and thinly sliced scallions.

variation

STIR-FRIED SALAD

For a warming-salad and stir-fry mashup, marinate only the cucumbers, scallions, and carrot, but don't marinate the cabbage. When you're ready to serve, heat a wok over high heat and drizzle with just a whisper of high-heat vegetable oil. Add the sliced cabbage and stir-fry less than 2 minutes, just enough to sear and slightly wilt the leaves. Empty the cabbage into a mixing bowl. Now stir-fry the cooked, chilled noodles, separating them into two batches. Add a little extra oil to keep from sticking and stir-fry only enough to sear. Serve noodles topped with the cabbage, marinated vegetables, and tofu.

KELP NOODLE PEKING TOFU SALAD

Omit the udon noodles. Prepare a package of kelp noodles by rinsing them with warm water and shaking them dry. Dress the noodles with a spoonful or two of vegetable pickling juices and assemble the salad.

KOREAN SHIITAKE BACON SALAD RICE BOWL

Makes 2 bowls

CHOOSE A DRESSING

Gochujang Dressing (recipe right here!)

Wasabi Miso Lime Dressing (page 56)

TOPPINGS—CHOOSE ONE TOFU AND/OR THE MAPLE MUSHROOM BACON

6 pieces Korean BBQ (page 86) or Sriracha Orange (page 90) or Savory Sesame Tamari (page 85) tofu, cut into thin slices

Maple Mushroom Bacon (page 125)

SALAD

3 cups cooked short-grain white or brown rice, kept warm

2 tablespoons rice vinegar

2 teaspoons agave nectar

½ teaspoon kosher salt

½ teaspoon toasted sesame oil

1 large carrot, peeled

½ pound daikon, peeled

½ pound spinach, thoroughly washed

2 cups cauliflower florets

1 tablespoon grape-seed oil

1 ripe Haas avocado, cut in half, peel and pit removed, halves thinly sliced

1 cup sunflower sprouts or microgreens

2 scallions, white and tender green parts, finely sliced

2 tablespoons black sesame seeds

1 sheet nori seaweed, cut into matchstick pieces

Bibimbap, the marvelous Korean dish of rice served with tidy portions of seasoned, lightly blanched fresh vegetables and a fiery, sweet red chile sauce, can be simulated at home. This casual Friday kind of rice bowl balances both raw and lightly blanched veggies, scattered atop hot rice, garnished with tasty toppings drenched with plenty of just-authentic-enough gochujang dressing, the secret sauce to the mouthwatering powers of bibimbap.

Prepare the tofu of choice and the mushroom bacon first; these can be prepared up to 2 days in advance.

When it's almost salad-serving time, make the rice and cover to keep warm. In a separate small bowl, whisk together the rice vinegar, agave, salt, and sesame oil.

Time to prepare those vegetables! Use the julienne blade on a mandoline to slice the carrot and daikon into matchsticks, and place each in a separate small bowl. Boil 1 quart of water and place the spinach in a colander in the sink. Pour the boiling water over the spinach to wilt; use long-handled tongs to stir the spinach around in the colander as you pour the water. Once the spinach is cool enough to handle, firmly squeeze handfuls to remove as much water as possible. Put the spinach in a small mixing bowl. Preheat the oven to 375°F, and on a small baking sheet, toss together cauliflower with grape-seed oil and, if desired, a pinch of kosher salt. Roast until tender, about 8 to 10 minutes, flipping once. Remove from oven and let cool while finishing rest of salad.

Continued

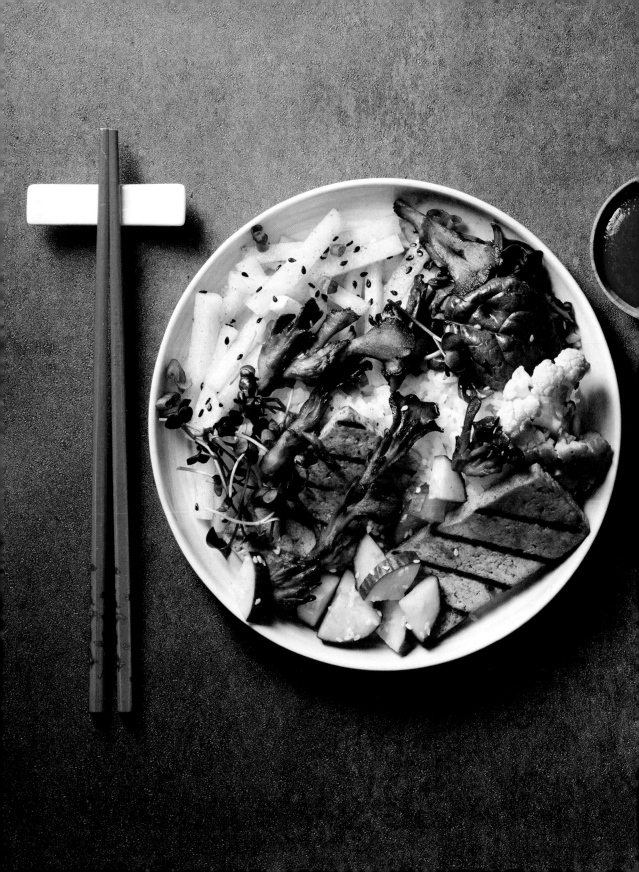

Pour a little of this vinegar dressing over the carrot and daikon, and use the remaining dressing to pour over the wilted spinach and cauliflower. Mix each veggie thoroughly to coat in the dressing.

Scoop warm rice into deep serving bowls. Arrange equal piles of carrot, daikon, spinach, and cauliflower on top of the rice. Add the tofu slices and the shiitake bacon, if using. Top with avocado, sprouts or microgreens, scallions, sesame seeds, and nori seaweed. Serve immediately with your dressing of choice!

GOCHUJANG DRESSING

¼ cup gochujang chile paste

⅓ cup warm water

1 teaspoon toasted sesame oil

The sublime Korean spicy sauce, made from fermented chile paste, becomes just a little more like a dressing just for salads. The essential ingredient is Korean gochujang, a dense, sweetened red chile paste that is spicy, but not searingly hot, and deeply flavorful. If you can't find gochujang paste, serve this salad with the Wasabi Miso Lime Dressing (page 56) and bring out a big bottle of sriracha sauce to pass around for anyone in need of a red chile fix.

Whisk all the ingredients together until smooth. Keep chilled until ready to serve and use within a day for the best flavor.

MUSTARD GREENS TABBOULEH WITH ALMONDS AND ROASTED CHICKPEAS

Serves 2 to 3

DRESSING

Maple Mustard Shallot Vinaigrette (page 70) or Pomegranate Vinaigrette (page 69)

TOPPING— CHOOSE ONE

Roasted Lemon Pepper Chickpeas (page 100)

6 cutlets of Tahini Miso tofu (page 92) or Savory Sesame Tamari tofu (page 85), diced

SALAD

1 tablespoon kosher salt

2 pounds mustard greens, washed and cut into 4-inch pieces

1 cup bulgur wheat, cooked according to the package directions

4 scallions, white parts and tender green parts, thinly sliced

1½ cups flat-leaf parsley, chopped, divided

½ cup mint, roughly chopped

1 small cucumber, peeled, seeded, and diced

1 pint cherry tomatoes, diced, or 2 medium red ripe tomatoes, seeded and diced

¼ cup slivered almonds, toasted

This is a tabbouleh (the classic Lebanese wheat and parsley salad) in spirit, but blanched and chopped mustard greens alongside parsley create a juicier, greener version with a spicy, earthy crunch. A bit of mustard and maple in the dressing take it a step or two further away from classic tabbouleh, but during hot, sweaty summer days, a bowl of this is light enough to cool you off but hearty enough to power you through the afternoon.

Why steamed mustard greens in a salad? Mustard greens, which are so good for vegan bones (lots of calcium), are underappreciated in most American cuisines. Cooked can have advantages over raw mustard; it tames the heat of spicy mustard greens (which can vary from variety to variety and the age and size of the leaves) and helps pack in more bone-building mustard greens per serving.

Roast the chickpeas or tofu first. While that's cooking, whisk the dressing of choice in a small bowl and keep chilled until ready to use.

Bring a 2-quart pot of water to boil over high heat, and fill another large bowl with cold water and keep it close by. Add a tablespoon of kosher salt to the boiling water, then add half of the mustard greens and blanch for about 30 seconds; the mustard leaves and stems will turn bright green. Use metal tongs or a spider skimmer to immediately transfer the greens to the bowl of cold water; this stops the

Continued

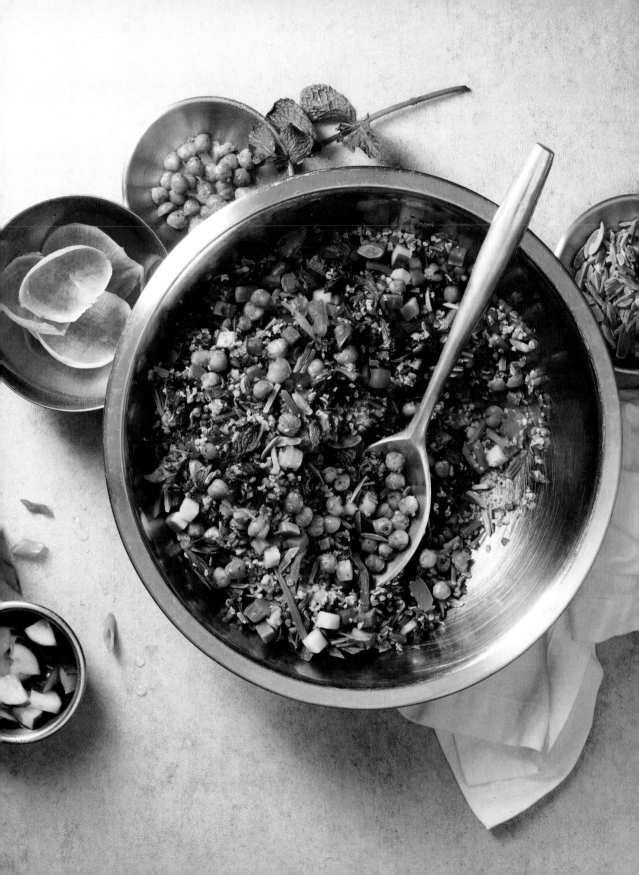

cooking process by cooling down the greens, keeping them firm and green yet tenderized by the quick dip in boiling water. Repeat with remaining greens. Drain the greens and gather in your hands to squeeze out excess water.

Finely chop the mustard greens and transfer to a mixing bowl. Add the cooked bulgur wheat, scallions, 1 cup chopped parsley, mint, cucumber, tomatoes, almonds, and half of the roasted chickpeas or diced tofu, and drizzle with half of the dressing. Combine thoroughly to coat with dressing. Scoop into a serving bowl, garnish with the remaining chickpeas and parsley, and drizzle with the rest of the dressing.

variation

GLUTEN-FREE

Substitute cooked red or multicolored quinoa blend for the bulgur wheat.

OTHER WHOLE-GRAIN WHEATS

Farro and freekeh (green, cracked sprouted wheat) are also great in this salad. Substitute cooked, cooled grain for the bulgur wheat.

PERUVIAN POTATO AND RED QUINOA SALAD

Serves 3 to 4

AJI AMARILLO DRESSING

1 garlic clove, peeled

1 teaspoon kosher salt

2 tablespoons lime juice

1 tablespoon white wine vinegar

1 tablespoon aji amarillo (yellow Peruvian chile) sauce, or 1 jalapeño pepper, half of the seeds removed and finely minced, plus a pinch of turmeric

2 teaspoons agave nectar

A few twists of freshly ground black pepper

¼ cup mild olive oil

TOPPING

½ cup Red Onion Quick Pickle (page 136)

4 to 6 cutlets of Peruvian Chile Lime roasted tofu (page 87), diced

SALAD

1 pound waxy (blue, Yukon Gold, or small red) potatoes

1 tablespoon kosher salt

1 cup cooked red quinoa

1 cup frozen corn kernels, rinsed with cool water to thaw

4 to 6 big lettuce leaves

1 cup cilantro, roughly chopped

½ cup chopped black olives

½ cup roasted peanuts, chopped

This beyond-the-pale of mayonnaise potato salad is seasoned with bright vinaigrette and garnished with the flavors of the homeland of potatoes, Peru: peanuts, cilantro, olives, a touch of cooked quinoa, and most Peruvian of all (but uncommon here still), aji amarillo, the marvelous yellow chile. Fresh aji amarillo is hard to come by in North America, but jars of easy-to-use golden yellow sauce made from these chiles is a common find in markets where Latin American groceries are sold. The usual substitution for aji amarillo is jalapeño peppers (about the same level of spiciness, or perhaps a little hotter); if you want to achieve the same yellow color, an optional pinch of turmeric will do the job.

In a 2-quart pot, cover the potatoes with 3 inches of water and stir in the salt. Bring to a rolling boil over high heat, then reduce the heat to medium and simmer the potatoes until fork tender, about 10 to 15 minutes. Immediately drain, and when cool to touch, dice the potatoes into bite-sized pieces. If using tiny potatoes, gently press potatoes with the back of a wooden spoon to crush slightly. In a mixing bowl, combine potatoes with diced tofu, quinoa, and corn.

Prepare the dressing; with a mortar and pestle, smash the garlic and salt into a paste. Scoop the paste into a small mixing bowl or large measuring cup, and add the remaining ingredients except the oil and whisk. Then drizzle the oil a little at a time, whisking until the mixture is smooth. Use promptly, as the dressing will naturally start to separate.

Continued

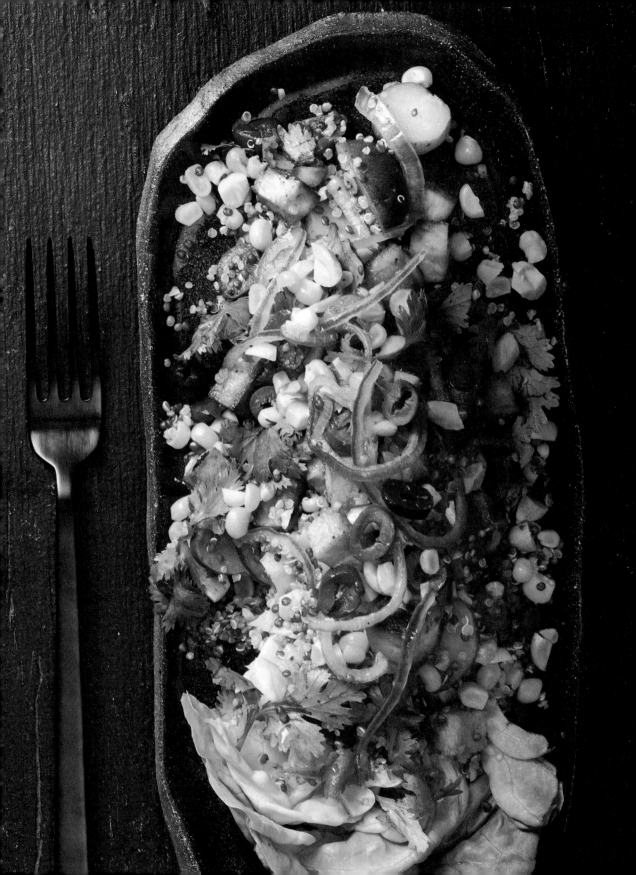

Drizzle half of the dressing over the potatoes and toss to coat. Arrange the lettuce leaves on a serving platter, and mound the potatoes over the leaves. Garnish with the pickled onions, cilantro, olives, and peanuts, and drizzle with the remaining dressing. Serve while the potatoes still have a touch of warmth.

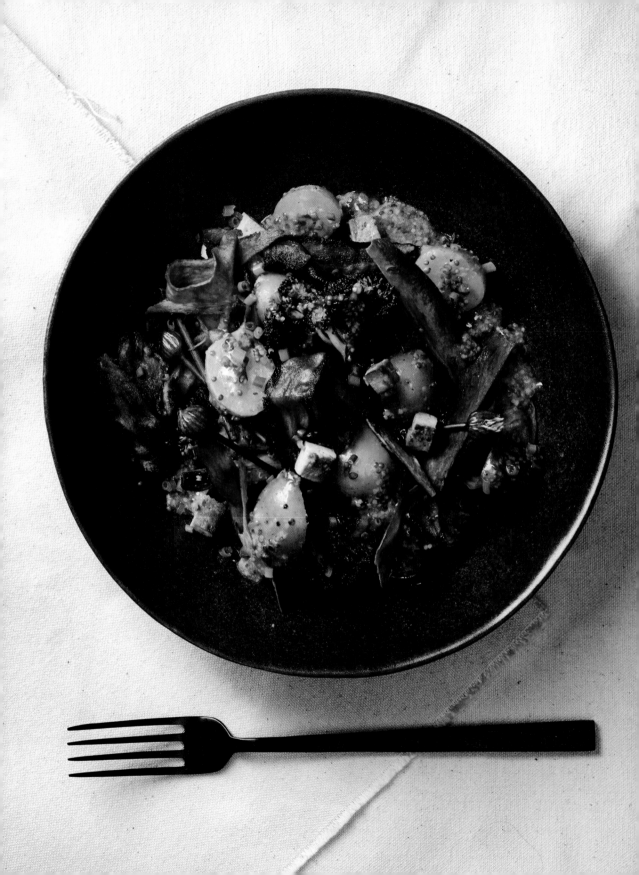

CHARRED BROCCOLI, POTATO, AND ROOT BACON SALAD

Serves 4

CHOOSE A DRESSING

Creamy Italian Hemp Dressing (page 33)

Hollyhock Dressing (page 61)

Maple Mustard Shallot Vinaigrette (page 70)

Oil-Free Cashew Lemon Pepper Dressing (page 46)

TOPPINGS

Maple Mushroom Bacon (page 125)

Root Bacon (page 127)

SALAD

1 pound broccoli

2 tablespoons olive oil

1 teaspoon kosher salt, plus additional salt, to taste

Freshly ground black pepper, to taste

1½ pounds red, yellow, or other waxy boiling potatoes

½ cup thinly sliced red onion

Potatoes and broccoli, a substantial vegetable love story forever. In this dressing-dappled instance, broccoli is seared in the oven and tossed with potatoes and vegan bacon for a boss salad that's a little like a deconstructed baked potato with the pub-grub vibes of the fully loaded potato skins. And don't limit yourself to just regular broccoli; tender, sweet broccolini or broccoli rabe are great in this salad too.

Charring the broccoli in the oven on a very hot preheated baking sheet is a convenient way to blacken a lot of broccoli all at once. If you prefer to prepare your broccoli in smaller batches, searing in a very hot cast-iron skillet on the stove top works just as well.

Prepare your choice of veggie bacon and/or Crispy, Cheesy Almond Crunch first. While the bacon is roasting, whisk the dressing of choice in a small bowl and keep chilled until ready to use.

Preheat the oven to 450°F, and slide a large baking sheet into the oven to preheat the sheet. Trim the stems from heads of broccoli and slice the broccoli heads into bite-sized pieces. Use a vegetable peeler to shave the tough outer skin from the stems, then dice the stems into ½-inch cubes. In a mixing bowl, toss the broccoli with the olive oil and rub the pieces thoroughly to coat evenly. Sprinkle salt and pepper over the broccoli.

Continued

While the oven preheats, dice the potatoes into 1-inch cubes. Transfer to a 2-quart soup pot and cover with 2 inches of cold water and stir in the teaspoon of salt. Bring to a boil over high heat, then reduce the heat to medium and simmer until the potatoes are tender but not falling apart, about 10 to 15 minutes. Drain and transfer to a large mixing bowl. Add the sliced onions to the bowl with the potatoes.

By now, the oven should blazing hot. Carefully remove the preheated sheet from the oven and scatter the oiled broccoli evenly over the sheet. Transfer the sheet back to the oven and roast, occasionally turning the broccoli pieces with a spatula or metal tongs until the broccoli is charred on the edges, about 5 to 8 minutes.

Add the charred broccoli and the sliced red onions to the potatoes. Drizzle half of the dressing over the veggies and gently toss to coat. Transfer to a large mixing bowl. Transfer the salad to individual serving plates or a serving platter or tray, and garnish as you like with veggie bacon and/or crispy, cheesy almonds. Serve pronto!

ROASTED TOMATO CHICKPEA PASTA SALAD

Serves 4

DRESSING

Balsamic Dijon
Vinaigrette
(page 71)

TOPPINGS

Caesar Walnuts
(page 123) or 1 cup
Kalamata olives,
pits removed

1 cup Roasted
Lemon Pepper
Chickpeas
(page 100)

SALAD

8 ounces chickpea
or other bean-
based pasta

4 cups chard
leaves, cut away
from the stems

2 tablespoons olive
oil, divided

1 pint cherry
tomatoes or grape
tomatoes

2 teaspoons
kosher salt, plus
more for sprinkling

Plenty of freshly
cracked black
pepper

½ cup sliced chard
stems

1 large red onion,
quartered and cut
into ¼-inch slices

1 cup basil leaves,
torn into bite-sized
pieces

I'm not the biggest pasta fan; if I'm going to eat flour for dinner, I want it to be tangy, whole-grain sourdough bread or a crusty baguette. But the recent wave of bean-based, naturally gluten-free pastas has me rethinking, and re-eating, that. Not only are these new-wave pastas loaded with protein and fiber, they taste fantastic. Chickpea-based pasta holds its own paired with flavorful dressings and roasted veggies. This simple salad is full of juicy flavors from roasted cherry tomatoes, savory Caesar Walnuts, Kalamata olives, or roasted chickpeas and chard prepared two ways.

Pasta salad should not be eaten ice cold out of the fridge; either serve it freshly made, or if it's your brown-bag lunch, gently warm it in the microwave for just 30 seconds or less to take off the chill.

Roast up the Caesar Walnuts or Roasted Lemon Pepper Chickpeas first. While the nuts or chickpeas are in the oven, whisk together the dressing.

Start cooking the pasta according to the package directions, using liberally salted water. While you wait for the water to boil, chiffonade the chard leaves, leaving the stems to the side. Wash the chard and spin dry and add to a large mixing bowl.

Cook the pasta until almost al dente, and just before you're ready to drain the pasta, toss in the chard leaves. Stir for 5 seconds to blanch the chard in the pasta water, then drain. Promptly rinse the pasta and veggies with cool water and shake to remove as much water as possible. Toss with 2 teaspoons of oil and set aside at room temperature.

Continued

I prefer lightly cooked chard to raw, but if you love raw chard, skip the blanching step and massage it with a dash of olive oil and salt.

Preheat the oven to 425°F, and line a large baking sheet with foil. Wash and pat dry the tomatoes and slice each in half. Arrange the tomatoes cut-side up on the foil and drizzle with a tablespoon or so of olive oil, then sprinkle with a healthy dash of kosher salt and black pepper. Slice the chard stems into ½-inch pieces. Slide the tomatoes into the oven and roast for 10 minutes; remove from the oven, push the tomatoes to one side of the baking sheet, and add the chard stems. Drizzle the chard stems with the remaining oil, sprinkle on some salt and pepper, and roast for another 10 minutes until the stems are tender and the tomatoes are sizzling. Remove from the oven.

Transfer the onion and basil leaves to a large mixing bowl. Add the roasted tomatoes and chard stems and then the cooked pasta and chard leaves. Add a tablespoon of dressing and toss to coat everything in dressing. Portion the pasta salad into individual servings, top with Caesar Walnuts or Kalamata olives and Roasted Lemon Pepper Chickpeas, and drizzle a little remaining dressing on and serve it up!

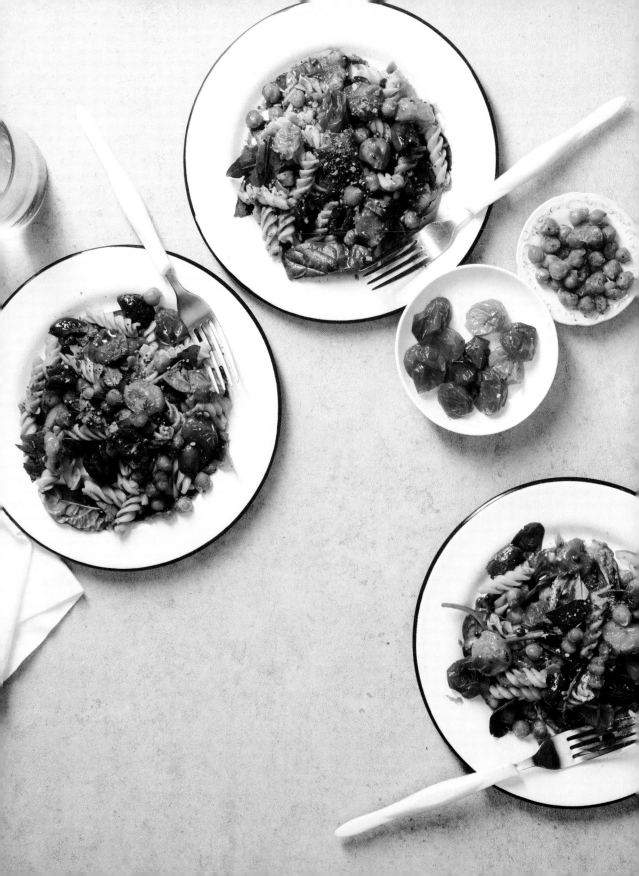

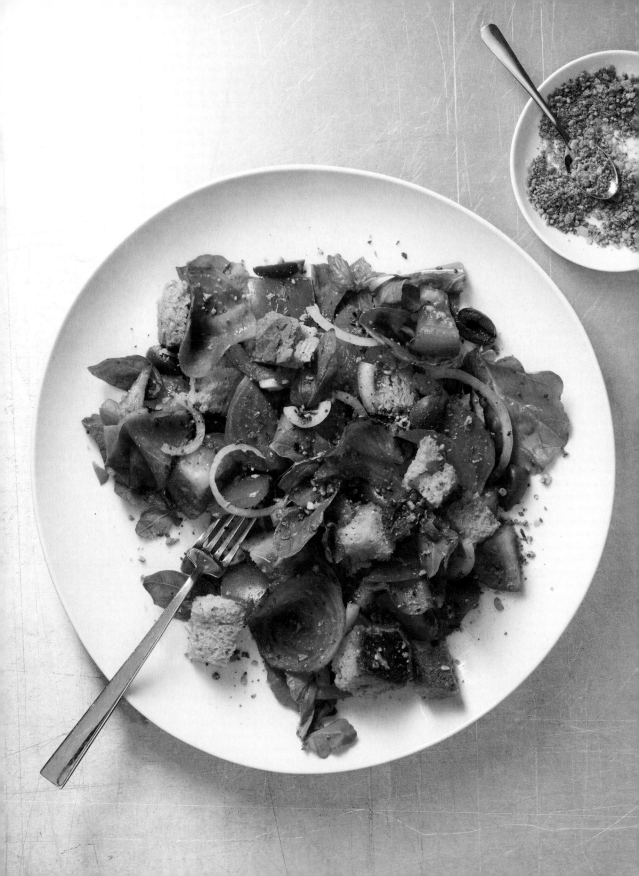

PIZZA PANZANELLA
WITH BEET PROSCIUTTO

Serves 3 to 4

TOPPINGS

1 cup or more Beet Prosciutto slices (page 131)

Naked Toasts (page 140)

½ cup Toasted Sun and Pepita Parm (page 110)

SALAD

3 pounds red, ripe, juicy summery tomatoes

3 garlic cloves, peeled

1 teaspoon kosher salt

2 tablespoons red wine vinegar

2 teaspoons dried oregano

½ teaspoon red pepper flakes

3 tablespoons good-quality extra-virgin olive oil

1 green bell pepper, seeds removed and diced

1 large red onion, quartered and cut into ¼-inch slices

1 cup Kalamata olives, pits removed

2 cups basil leaves, large leaves torn into bite-sized pieces

2 cups baby arugula

Do you have so many big, juicy, bursting-with-flavor summer heirloom tomatoes that you're paying people to haul them away from you? Well, I never do, but when that day comes, this summertime salad will save the day. This salad must be made with prime in-season tomatoes! They are so naturally juicy and flavorful they practically make their own dressing for panzanella, that Tuscan salad of transforming day-old bread into an outrageously fresh tomato salad. With a few pizza toppings thrown into the breezy warm-weather salad, it doesn't get better than this!

Prepare the Beet Prosciutto, Naked Toasts, and Toasted Sun and Pepita Parm first. You can do all of this up to 3 days (or a month for the croutons) in advance and keep chilled or stored until showtime!

Remove the cores from the tomatoes, then dice the tomatoes, making sure to save as much as the runny juices as possible. I often dice very juicy tomatoes on a large dinner plate just to save those juices, but a flexible cutting board can also do the job. Pour the juices into a large mixing bowl.

With a mortar and pestle, pound the garlic cloves and salt together into a creamy paste. Scoop the paste into the mixing bowl with the tomato juices and whisk in the vinegar, oregano, pepper flakes, and oil. Fold in the tomatoes, bell pepper, onion, and olives. Cover and chill the bowl for an hour to marinate the tomatoes and blend the flavors.

Continued

A few minutes before serving, fold in the naked croutons and the basil leaves. To serve, scoop the panzanella into a serving bowl. Make sure to pour any remaining juices from the mixing bowl over the salad and garnish top with folded slices of Beet Prosciutto, arugula, and a generous dusting of Toasted Sun and Pepita Parm. *Mangia!*

ZUCCHINI AND CHICKPEA FATTOUSH SALAD

Serves 2 to 3

CHOOSE A DRESSING

Pomegranate Vinaigrette (page 69)

Oregano Garlic Lemon Vinaigrette (page 69)

SALAD

2 whole-wheat or white pita bread

¼ section of Salted Lemon rind (page 64), minced (optional but perfect here)

1 young (8-inch) zucchini, diced

1 small cucumber, preferably Persian or hothouse cucumber, peeled, seeded, and diced

2 large ripe tomatoes, diced

½ cups cooked chickpeas, well rinsed

2 scallions, white and green parts, thinly sliced

1 cup chopped parsley

4 cups chopped romaine lettuce

½ cup chopped cilantro

2 tablespoons chopped mint

3 tablespoons pomegranate arils

1 tablespoon sumac powder, if desired

Fattoush is yet another amazing bread salad; the crunchy contrast of cucumber and pita with juicy, herby tomatoes makes this a refreshing warm-weather entrée salad. The unconventional addition of chickpeas, young, tender zucchini, and even some romaine lettuce makes this yet another well-rounded meal of a salad. Live above a pita bakery and get fresh-baked pita daily? Then this is your new favorite recipe to use up day-old pita. For everyone else who must get pita bread from the supermarket, the easy-to-find, straight-out-of-the-package pita is fine anytime.

Whisk the dressing ingredients together in a small bowl and chill until ready to use. Preheat the oven to 375°F and pull apart each pita along the seams into two halves. Place on a baking sheet and toast the pita halves for about 10 to 12 minutes until crisp and dry. Break the pita into bite-sized pieces.

In a large mixing bowl, combine the dressing with the salted lemon rind, zucchini, cucumber, tomatoes, and chickpeas. Cover and chill in the refrigerator for 30 minutes or up to an hour to marinate.

When you're ready for the fattoush, add to the zucchini mixture the scallions, parsley, cilantro, lettuce, mint, and pomegranate arils and stir to combine. Add the pita and stir again, then mound the salad into a serving bowl or individual servings. Sprinkle with sumac powder, if using, and serve at once.

Continued

tip

The key to tenderizing and pumping flavor into mellow summer squash is to set it aside to marinade in the acidic dressing first, then add it to the salad just before serving.

Pomegranate molasses is the richly flavored result of boiling down pomegranate juice to a thick, rich syrup with an intense sweet-sour fruity flavor. If you can't find pomegranate molasses for the dressing (Mediterranean grocery stores and even some Whole Foods stock it now), just leave it out. There's really no substitute (and please don't use regular sugarcane molasses).

variation

FATTOUSH NOW AND LATER

Fattoush is a fantastic salad to prepare in advance, up to 24 hours, and have a batch on hand for dinner tonight and lunch tomorrow. Store the prepared salad, minus the toasted pita pieces, in a container in the fridge. Store the pita in an airtight container on the countertop. For each serving of fattoush, scoop out a heaping cup of salad, add a big handful of toasted pita, combine, and serve with a sprinkle of sumac.

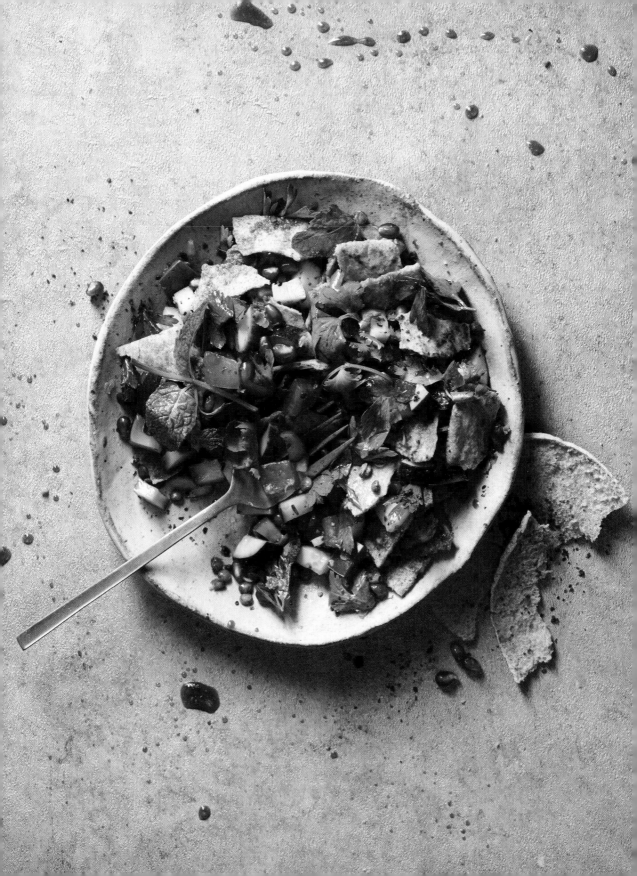

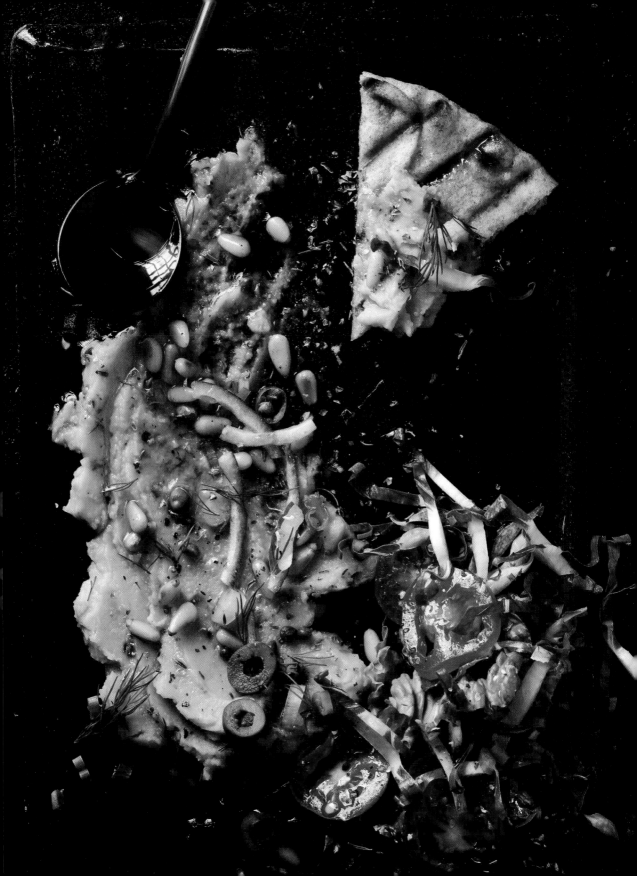

GREEK GOLDEN
FAVA SALAD PITA

Serves 4 to 6

FAVA SPLIT PEA SPREAD

¼ cup olive oil

3 garlic cloves, chopped, about 1 heaping tablespoon

½ cup diced red onion or shallots

1 cup uncooked yellow split peas

1 bay leaf

1½ teaspoons kosher salt

2 scallions, sliced thin

FOR THE PITA

4 to 6 thick, no-pocket Greek-style pita or gluten-free flatbread

Good quality extra-virgin olive oil

1 pound ripe tomatoes, sliced thin

1 red onion, sliced paper thin

1 large cucumber, seeds removed and sliced thin

Big handful of romaine lettuce or radicchio

½ cup Kalamata olives, pits removed and sliced

¼ cup toasted pine nuts

Crumbly, Salty Almond Cheese (page 113) or prepared vegan feta cheese (optional)

Fava is simple, wholesome Greek meze, a simply seasoned spread of yellow split peas. Creamy and tasty warm or cold, it could very well be the next hummus. Or at least something to eat on your days off of hummus eating.

There are a few ways to make fava, most involving simmering yellow split peas with onions and garlic, then blending the cooked mash with plenty of olive oil for a rich texture. Don't forget to be a little generous with the kosher salt; bean dishes really need the extra zing of proper seasoning to pull together their starchy, mild texture and flavor.

Once chilled, fava firms up considerably. It's almost sliceable, making it an interesting pâté-like topping on salads or sliced for sandwiches, but it's soft enough to mash with a fork and slather over toast. While it's a spread, one of the best ways in my opinion is to enjoy it piled with salad: tomatoes, cucumbers, onions, even grilled greens (or fresh), and of course, pita.

In a 2-quart saucepan, add the oil and fry the garlic and onion or shallots over low heat. Fry for 10 minutes, stirring occasionally, until the vegetables are pale golden and tender.

Rinse split peas and add to the saucepan. Add 2½ cups of water, bay leaf, and salt. Bring to a rolling boil, skim off the foam, and partially cover. Reduce the heat to medium-low and simmer for 30 minutes, or until peas are soft and no hard centers remain. Remove and discard the bay leaf.

Continued

variation——

JUST THE FAVA

To serve, spread the fava into a thick, swirly layer in the serving dish. Drizzle with olive oil, sprinkle with coarse salt and cracked pepper, or if you like, sprinkle with some minced scallions or dried oregano. Serve with crusty bread or grilled pita.

Once the peas are tender, add the scallions and simmer another 2 minutes. Turn off the heat and pulse with an immersion blender into a thick purée. Spoon into a serving dish, or into a storage container and chill until just ready to serve.

Preheat a cast-iron pan or cast-iron grill pan over high heat. Brush pita with oil. Grill on the hot cast-iron pan, flipping once, for about 2 minutes, or until the bread is hot and softened.

For the final presentation, spread a thick layer of the fava spread over the hot pita, layer with the vegetables and greens, sprinkle with the olives, pine nuts, and almond cheese, if using. Drizzle with olive oil, slice into wedges, and eat!

AVOCADO AND BLACK BEAN SALAD ON CORNBREAD TOAST

Makes 4

DRESSING

Tahini Mayo
(page 43)

UNDERNEATH THE SALAD

4 (1-inch-thick) slices of Vegan Cornbread Loaf (page 146)

SALAD

2 tablespoons lime juice

¼ teaspoon chipotle pepper powder

½ teaspoon kosher salt

A few twists of black pepper

1 cup diced, juicy summery tomatoes or diced wintery grape tomatoes

1 cup cooked black beans, drained and rinsed

½ cup fresh corn kernels or thawed frozen corn

1 medium red onion, quartered and cut into ¼-inch slices

1 scallion, white and tender green parts, minced

½ cup roughly chopped cilantro, plus 2 tablespoons for garnish

½ cup roughly chopped basil or dill

Olive oil, for drizzling

1 large, ripe Haas avocado, halved and pit removed

Extra lime juice, about a tablespoon, for drizzling

Smoked sweet paprika, for sprinkling

Chipotle pepper–laced black bean corn salad loaded with avocado. Big slabs of toasted homemade vegan cornbread. A garlicky olive oil, a smear of buttery Tahini Mayo (page 43), a dusting of smoked paprika. An evolution in avocado toast. Or maybe a radical, tasty mutation!

Not some dainty, new-age day-spa avo toast—this is knife-and-fork, dinner-plate, roll-up-your-sleeves kind of avocado toast. As the cornbread must be toasted, it also needs to be baked in advance (it's best if it's a day old too), but you can plan accordingly by making the mayo and salad, without the diced avocado, a day in advance and storing it in the fridge too.

Bake and cool the Vegan Cornbread Loaf; day-old cornbread is ideal for toast. Whip up the Tahini Mayo and chill until ready to use.

In a mixing bowl, whisk together the lime juice, chipotle powder, salt, and pepper. Add the tomatoes, beans, corn, red onion, scallion, cilantro, and basil or dill. Toss the ingredients together, cover, and chill for 10 minutes.

Preheat a cast-iron skillet over medium-high heat. Drizzle a little oil over the cornbread and toast the slabs in the pan, two at time, until each side is lightly browned. For best results flip once, after each side has nicely toasted. Transfer toasts to serving dishes.

Continued

Thinly slice each avocado half and fan out on the cutting board. Portion out ½ of each fan for each toast. Spread each toast with a generous schmear of Tahini Mayo. Divide the corn and bean salad and top each toast, followed by a quarter fan of avocado.

Drizzle the oil and the lime juice on each toast, sprinkle with the smoked paprika, and top with a little extra cilantro. Serve right away with a knife and fork! And probably some napkins and, if you still insist, some Enya playing gently in the background.

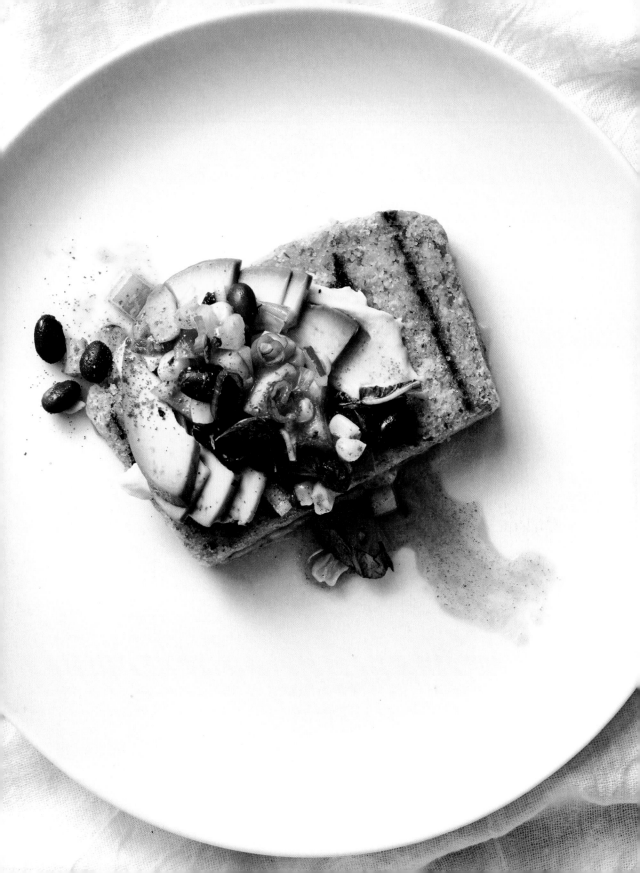

Soup and salad. Fire and ice. Darkness and light. Winter and summer. While seemingly from different parts of the kitchen, these two everyday meal mainstays have so much in common. Both are pillars of cuisine and comforting ways to eat some of the healthiest of foods—vegetables, legumes, even grains—and full of creative potential.

When soup and salad join forces, we all win a satisfying meal packed with good-for-you veggies and plant-based proteins. The following recipes opt for putting a small salad on top of your soup. Yes. Soup under salad. Salad on soup. Don't put down the book just yet . . . the contrast of warm soup and crunchy cool salad is a discovery of cool comfort. Still too out there? Opt to make a double batch of salad and serve it on the side, or before, or after the soup (so French!) for a crisp palate cleanser.

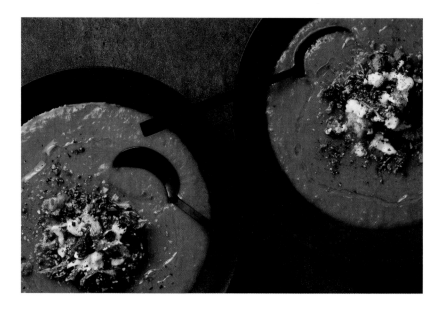

POTATO LEEK SOUP WITH BROCCOLI GREMOLATA

Serves 4 generously

POTATO LEEK SOUP

2 tablespoons vegan butter or olive oil

2 shallots, peeled and diced

1 large leek, white and tender light green parts only, cleaned and thinly sliced

2 pounds starchy white potatoes, unpeeled and diced

6 cups vegetable broth

1 teaspoon dried thyme or herbes de Provence

1 teaspoon kosher salt

Freshly ground black pepper, to taste

BROCCOLI GREMOLATA

¼ cup slivered almonds

Grated zest of 1 lemon, or ½ (2 sections) Salted Lemon rind (page 64)

2 tablespoons lemon juice

2 garlic cloves, peeled and minced

1 tablespoon olive oil

1 teaspoon kosher salt

2 cups shredded broccoli stems (such as broccoli slaw) or 3 cups broccoli florets

½ cup roughly chopped flat-leaf parsley

Creamy potato leek soup is made even better with broccoli. Here, this favorite cruciferous veggie gets a makeover. Broccoli florets (or even better, the crisp, sweet stems) are chopped for a more substantial twist on gremolata, a zippy, crunchy, and refreshing minced relish of parsley, lemon zest, garlic, and nuts.

In place of broccoli, try out broccolini, Chinese broccoli, or even kale stems or collard stems. Any substantial cruciferous vegetable stem can play well in this topping. You can also challenge the potato; starchy Russet types are expected, but waxy yellow Yukons or reds are excellent. Notice the potatoes remain unpeeled in this soup; I love the rustic bits of skin in the soup, but for something a little more sophisticated, do go ahead and peel 'em.

In a 2-quart soup pot over medium-low heat, melt the vegan butter and stir in the shallots and leek. Fry until the shallots and leek are very tender but before they can brown, about 6 to 8 minutes. Add the potatoes, broth, thyme, salt, and pepper.

Increase the heat to medium-high and bring the soup to a rapid simmer for 10 minutes, then reduce the heat to low and partially cover. Simmer the soup for another 10 to 15 minutes, or until the potatoes are very tender.

Use an immersion blender to pulse the soup into an almost smooth mixture (some tiny lumps are okay).

Continued

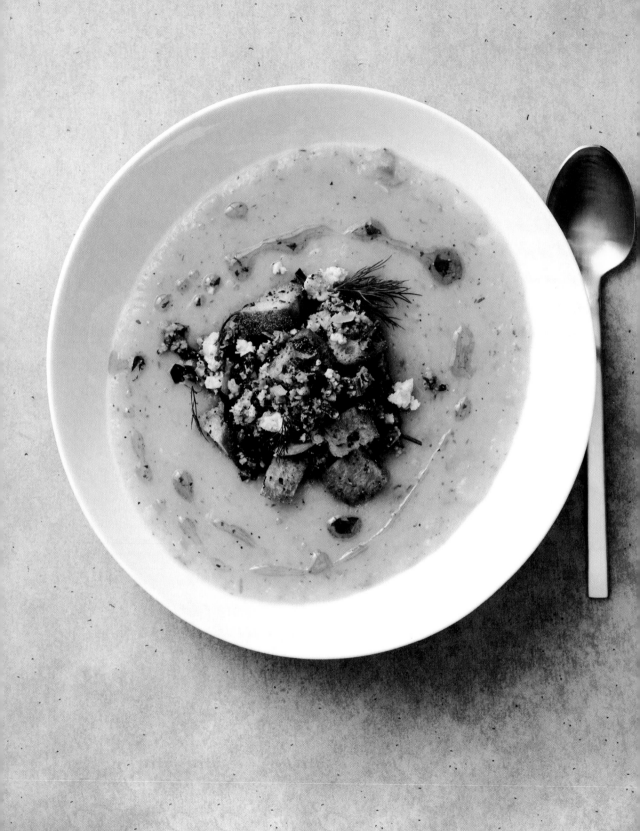

Taste the soup and season with a pinch or two more salt. Turn off the heat and cover the soup; let it rest while you prepare the salad.

In a food processor, roughly chop the almonds. Add the lemon zest, lemon juice, garlic, oil, and salt and pulse a few more times. Add the broccoli stems or florets and parsley. Pulse only a few times to finely chop the stems; don't overprocess or you may accidently end up with a moist paste (something that looks like broccoli hummus). The gremolata is ready when the broccoli is thoroughly chopped and the mixture is evenly combined.

Divide the soup into serving bowls and top with a heaping tablespoon or two of gremolata. Serve immediately and use the gremolata within a day of preparing!

Tip

FIX THAT LEEK

Lovely leeks usually hide a fair amount of sand or grit tucked in their leaves. There are a few traditional ways to clean leeks—most of them involving slicing down the center lengthwise and soaking in water. But if leeks are going to be diced for soup, my preferred method is to trim and dice the leeks first, dump them into a large metal mesh colander, then rinse them well under running water. Fast and no extra bowl required.

BUFFALO TOMATO SOUP WITH KALE CAESAR SALAD

Serves 4

BUFFALO TOMATO SOUP

2 tablespoons vegan butter or olive oil

2 shallots, peeled and minced

1 medium yellow onion, peeled and diced

½ teaspoon celery seed

1 (28-ounce) can diced fire-roasted tomatoes

3 cups vegetable broth

2 heaping tablespoons tomato paste

½ teaspoon kosher salt

2 to 3 tablespoons Frank's RedHot sauce or similar vinegar-based hot sauce

Freshly ground black pepper to taste

KALE CAESAR SALAD

2 to 3 tablespoons Hemp Seed Caesar Dressing (page 31)

Toasted Sun and Pepita Parm (page 110)

3 cups kale, torn into bite-sized pieces

½ cup shredded carrot or thinly sliced celery

2 cups Cheesy, Crispy Croutons (page 142) or croutons of your choice (pages 137–145)

This pantry-ready tomato soup is infused with tangy hot sauce and garnished with cool and zesty kale Caesar salad. Top with plenty of Cheesy, Crispy Croutons (page 142) and cheesy, nutty grated "parm" for that essential cheesy touch. Looking for a soup that feels like Saturday night pub grub but is sensible enough for a post-workday Tuesday night? Here you go.

Prepare the Hemp Seed Caesar Dressing and Toasted Sun and Pepita Parm first, and keep chilled until ready to use.

In a 2-quart soup pot over medium heat, melt the vegan butter and stir in the shallots and onion. Fry until the onion is soft and transparent, about 5 minutes, then stir in the celery seed and fry for 30 seconds. Add the entire can—juices and all—of the tomatoes, broth, tomato paste, salt, hot sauce, and black pepper.

Bring the soup to a rapid simmer for 5 minutes, then reduce the heat and simmer another 5 minutes. Use an immersion blender to pulse the soup into a smooth mixture. Turn off the heat and cover the soup; let it rest while you prepare the salad. In a mixing bowl, toss together the Caesar salad ingredients, making sure to coat the croutons with dressing as well.

Ladle the soup into generous-sized soup bowls and top with a generous cup of salad. Sprinkle with Toasted Sun and Pepita Parm and serve.

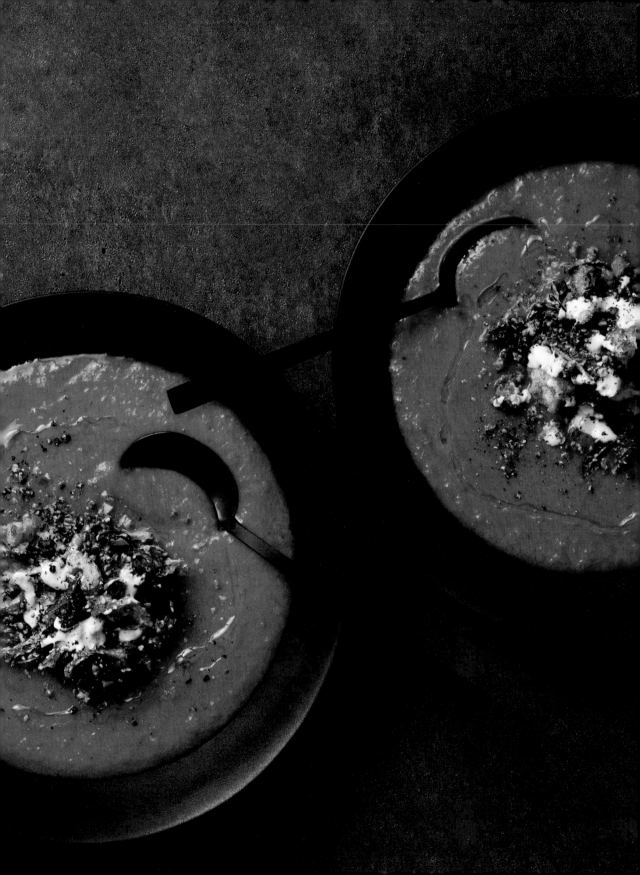

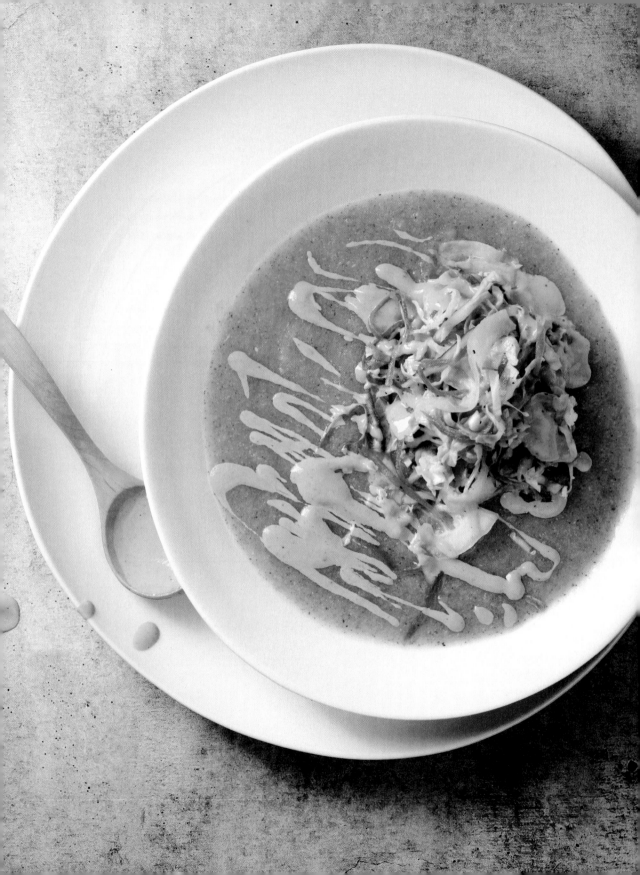

GREEN AGAIN SOUP
WITH TAHINI MISO SLAW

Serves 4 to 6

GREEN AGAIN SOUP

2 tablespoons olive oil

1-inch-thick piece of fresh ginger, peeled and diced

1 medium yellow onion, peeled and diced

1 large leek, white and tender light green parts only, cleaned and thinly sliced

2 cups cauliflower florets, chopped

1 pound baby bok choy, chopped, or 3 cups kale, chopped

1 green apple, unpeeled, seeds removed, and diced

6 cups vegetable broth

1 teaspoon kosher salt

½ teaspoon dried thyme

1 cup chopped parsley or cilantro

Freshly ground black pepper

TAHINI MISO SLAW

Turmeric Tahini Miso Sauce (page 44)

4 ounces Brussels sprouts, shredded

2 scallions, white and tender green parts, thinly sliced

1 orange or red carrot, julienned

1 teaspoon minced Salted Lemon rind (page 64) or ½ teaspoon grated lemon zest

What every lover of vegan junk food needs in between the vegan doughnuts, vegan pizza, and dairy-free ice cream that our bold new vegan world has to offer: a smooth soup packed with all manner of healthy green veggies, a bit of fruit, and plenty of fresh herbs.

Topped with golden tahini–dressed, shredded Brussels sprouts, this lovely jade-green soup is a compact way to get in all the greens any time of the year, again and again, but really rewarding during the cool winter months with their heavy, starchy foods.

In a 2-quart soup pot over medium heat, heat the oil and stir in the ginger, onion, and leek. Fry until the onion and leek are very soft but before they can brown, about 5 minutes. Add the cauliflower, bok choy, apple, broth, and the salt.

Increase the heat to medium and bring the soup to a gentle simmer for 10 minutes, then reduce the heat to low, add the thyme, and partially cover. Simmer the soup for another 5 minutes, or until the cauliflower is very tender, then add parsley or cilantro and black pepper.

Use an immersion blender to pulse the soup into a silky-smooth mixture. Taste the soup and season with a pinch or two more salt. Turn off the heat and cover the soup; let it rest while you prepare the salad.

In a mixing bowl, fold ¼ cup of Turmeric Tahini Miso Sauce with the shredded sprouts, scallions, carrot and lemon rind.

Divide the soup into serving bowls and top with a cup of slaw. Drizzle on some additional Turmeric Tahini Miso Sauce and sip your veggies!

CREAMY CAULIFLOWER SOUP WITH APPLE WALNUT SALAD

Serves 4

CREAMY CAULIFLOWER SOUP

2 tablespoons olive oil

1 shallot, peeled and chopped

2 cups diced white onion

1 cup diced peeled parsnip

1½ pounds (8-inch head) cauliflower florets

6 cups vegetable broth

1 teaspoon dried thyme

1½ teaspoons kosher salt, plus more, to taste

2 tablespoons nutritional yeast

2 teaspoons white wine vinegar

Freshly cracked black pepper, to taste

APPLE WALDORF SALAD

1 tablespoon lemon juice

2 teaspoons grapeseed oil

½ teaspoon mustard powder

½ teaspoon kosher salt

1 cup diced unpeeled apple

1 cup diced celery

½ cup walnut halves, toasted and coarsely chopped

½ cup chopped flat-leaf parsley

A few healthy twists of freshly ground black pepper

Silken and creamy cauliflower soup, with sweetness from sautéed onions and parsnips and a hint of umami from nooch, is yet another way to eat everyone's new favorite vegetable. Puréed cauliflower soup is elegant as is, but it gets the highbrow tennis-club treatment topped with a lighter, tangier version of Waldorf salad. Historically, this apple-celery-walnut salad is dressed with mayo, but I prefer a clean lemon vinaigrette. Crisp, cool, and a little fruity, this classy salad displayed on top of the cream-colored soup is sure to be the talk of your next country-club soirée or just tastes pretty special eaten in your gym shorts while watching some tennis on your phone.

In a 2-quart soup pot over medium heat, heat the oil until it shimmers. Add the shallot and onion, stir and partially cover. Fry until soft and translucent, about 3 minutes, then stir in the parsnip, cover again, and fry for 3 to 4 minutes until the bits are slightly soft. Add the cauliflower, broth, thyme, and salt.

Increase the heat to medium-high and bring the soup to a rapid simmer for 5 minutes, then reduce the heat to low and partially cover. Simmer the soup for another 15 to 20 minutes, or until the cauliflower is very tender.

Add the nutritional yeast and vinegar, and use an immersion blender to pulse the soup into a smooth mixture. Taste the broth and season with a pinch or two

Continued

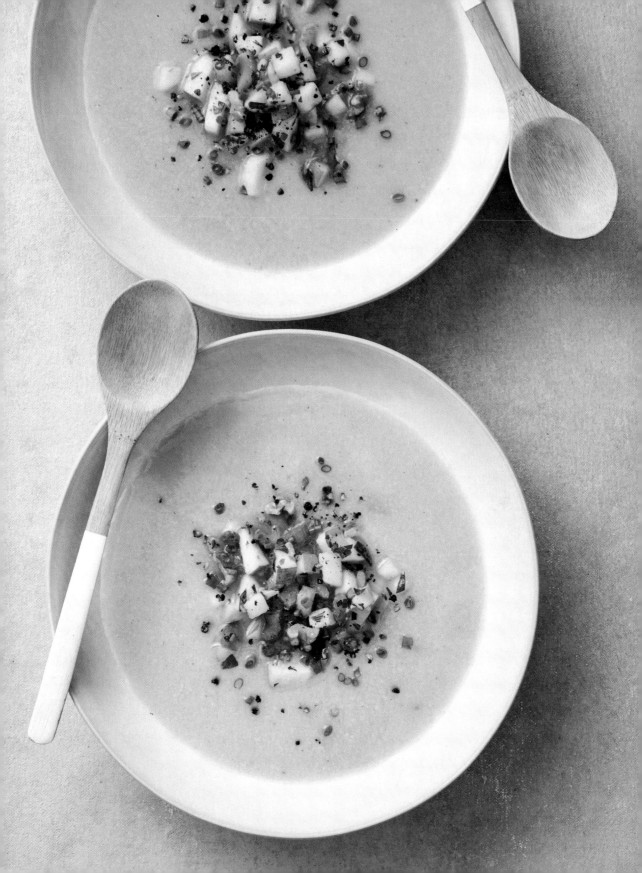

more salt and pepper, or a dash of white wine vinegar or an additional spoonful of nutritional yeast if necessary. Turn off the heat and cover the soup; let it rest while you prepare the salad.

In a mixing bowl, whisk together the lemon juice, oil, mustard powder, and salt until smooth. Fold in the apple, celery, walnuts, and parsley. Season with the black pepper and a dash of salt as desired.

Divide the soup into serving bowls and top with a scoop of salad and perhaps another dusting of black pepper and serve hot!

ETHIOPIAN RED LENTILS WITH BUTTERNUT AND AVOCADO COLLARD SALAD

Serves 4

ETHIOPIAN RED LENTILS WITH BUTTERNUT

1 pound butternut squash, seeds removed, peeled, and cubed

4 tablespoons olive oil, divided

1 large yellow onion, peeled and minced

2 garlic cloves, peeled and minced

2-inch piece ginger, peeled and minced

½ teaspoon ground turmeric

½ teaspoon ground cumin

2½ teaspoons berbere spice blend

1 cup red lentils, rinsed

1 teaspoon kosher salt

1 tablespoon lemon juice

½ cup chopped cilantro

1 lemon, quartered

Additional olive oil, for drizzling

AVOCADO COLLARD SALAD

1 garlic clove

½ teaspoon kosher salt

2 tablespoons lime juice

2 teaspoons olive oil

Big pinch cayenne pepper

4 large collard leaves, stems removed

1 ripe Haas avocado, pit removed, peeled and diced

Inspired by the wonderful Ethiopian dish messer wot, this rich red lentil soup is enriched with roasted butternut squash, then topped with a refreshing avocado and collard greens salad. Substitute sugar pumpkin or your favorite winter squash when it's in season, or try tropical pumpkin varieties such as calabaza. If you're lucky enough to have real injera to scoop up the soup, try it out, but a side of whole-wheat couscous or even naan tastes just as good. For authentic Ethiopian flavor, you'll need to locate berbere spice blend, a more common find in better gourmet markets (or Ethiopian groceries, if you have one nearby) with the growing popularity of Ethiopian food.

Preheat the oven to 400°F and line a baking sheet with parchment paper or foil. Pile the squash cubes in the center of the sheet, drizzle 2 tablespoons of oil over the squash, and toss the cubes to coat. Sprinkle with a big pinch of salt and spread in a single layer. Roast for 25 to 30 minutes, stirring occasionally, until the cubes are tender and brown. Remove from the oven and set aside.

While the squash roasts, heat the remaining oil in a 2-quart soup pot over medium heat. Stir in the onion, garlic, and ginger and fry for 3 minutes, or until the onion is very soft but not browned. Stir in the spices and the lentils, then pour in 4 cups of water and the salt. Increase the heat to high and bring the lentils to a rapid simmer for 3 minutes. Reduce the heat to low, partially cover, and

Continued

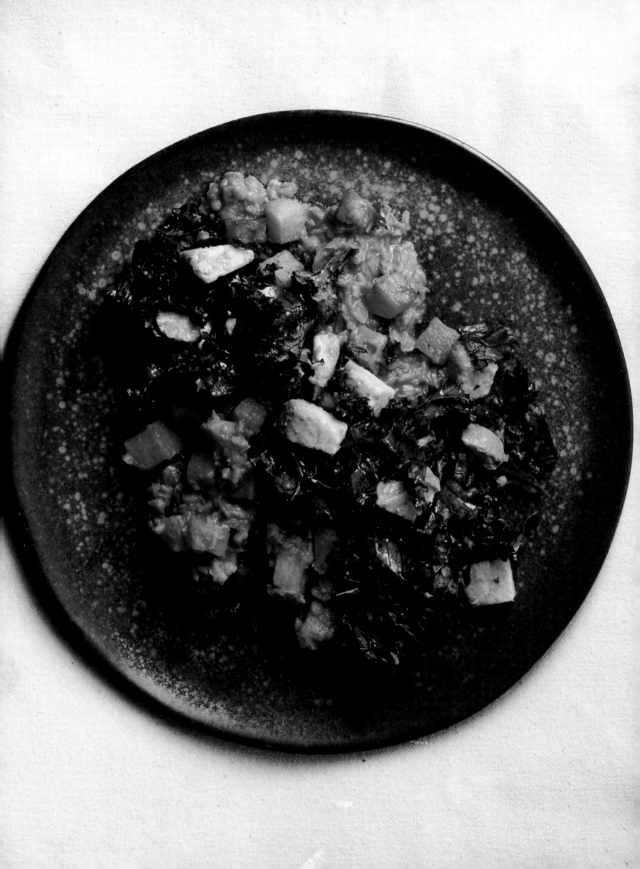

simmer the lentils for 35 to 40 minutes, or until the lentils are very tender and have melted down into a rich stew. Stir occasionally. If the mixture seems too thick and stiff, pour in ½ cup of water and simmer until done, then turn off the heat.

Stir in the roasted squash, lemon juice, and chopped cilantro. Taste and adjust the seasonings with salt and lemon juice if necessary. Cover and prepare the salad (if you didn't already while the stew was simmering!).

In a mortar and pestle, crush the garlic with the salt. Scoop the garlic into a mixing bowl and stir in the lime juice, oil, and cayenne. Stack the collards and roll them into a tight cigar, then slice the roll into thin strips. Add to the dressing mixture and massage the collards into the dressing for a minute or two until the collards have tenderized a bit and are shiny. Fold in the diced avocado.

Serve the stew in shallow bowls, spreading it in an even layer on the bottom of the bowl. Arrange the salad on top of the stew and squeeze a lemon wedge over the salad and drizzle some olive oil, if desired. Serve with injera bread (Ethiopian teff crepes), hot couscous, or crusty bread.

BABY CARROT GINGER SOUP WITH SESAME SLAW

Serves 4

BABY CARROT GINGER SOUP

1 pound baby carrots or just over 1 pound "adult" carrots

1 medium (8-ounce) orange sweet potato, scrubbed and diced

2 tablespoons olive oil or virgin coconut oil

2 large shallots, peeled and chopped

1 tablespoon minced ginger

1 teaspoon mild or hot curry powder

4 cups vegetable broth

½ teaspoon kosher salt

SESAME SLAW

1-inch-thick slice of peeled ginger

2 garlic cloves

1 tablespoon white miso

2 tablespoons lemon juice

1 tablespoon toasted sesame seeds

1 tablespoon olive oil

2 teaspoons toasted sesame oil

3 cups thinly sliced napa cabbage

½ cup chopped cilantro

Carrots and cabbage are reliably good produce finds year-round in most average grocery stores—which means you can whip up this fast, warming, spicy combo when winter winds are howling at your door. And if that's not easy enough, the sweet and soothing carrot ginger soup is made with the help of an everyday bag of baby carrots: nothing to peel, perfectly portioned into 1-pound bags. The sesame-dressed cabbage salad is a warming and yet cool, crunchy complement to the ginger soup. There's no better way to get a healthy veggie soup on a weeknight. (Of course, it's entirely possible to prepare this with "adult" carrots, and while these carrots will require slicing, regular carrots are often fresher and better tasting. I give you options!)

Remove the baby carrots from their bag, dump them into a colander, and rinse. Shake dry and dice the carrots into 1-inch pieces (if using adult carrots, scrub and dice into 1-inch pieces). Scrub the sweet potato (no need to peel) and dice into 1-inch cubes. In a 2-quart soup pot over medium heat, heat the oil for 15 seconds, then stir in the shallot and ginger. Sauté for about 1½ minutes to soften up the shallot, then stir in the carrots and sweet potato.

Fry the vegetables for another 2 minutes, then sprinkle in the curry powder and fry another 30 seconds. Pour in the broth and salt and increase the heat to high. Bring to a gentle boil, then lower the heat to medium-low and simmer for 12 to 15 minutes, or until the carrots and potatoes are tender. Reduce the heat to low and use an immersion blender to pulse the soup until completely smooth and creamy. Taste and, if you like, season with a little more salt, freshly ground pepper, or a dash of lime juice. Turn off the heat and cover the soup until ready to serve.

While the soup simmers, in a mortar and pestle, pound together the ginger, garlic, and miso into a paste. Transfer to a large mixing bowl and use a wire whisk to mix in the lemon juice, sesame seeds, olive oil, and sesame oil. Add the cabbage and cilantro and use long-handled tongs to thoroughly toss the ingredients together and coat everything in dressing. Cover the salad bowl and keep chilled until ready to serve.

Ready to eat? Ladle the soup into generous serving bowls and top with a hearty portion of salad, about 1 cup per bowl, and serve immediately.

CRANBERRY BEAN AND PASTA STEW WITH FENNEL SLAW

Serves 8

CRANBERRY BEAN AND PASTA STEW

16 ounces dry cranberry beans

4 garlic cloves, chopped

3 teaspoons kosher salt, plus more for sprinkling

¼ cup olive oil

1 large white onion, peeled and diced

2 celery stalks, diced

2 bay leaves

1 teaspoon ground cumin

¼ teaspoon cayenne pepper or ½ teaspoon hot pepper flakes

1 cup small pasta shapes (such as tiny shells or macaroni), uncooked

Freshly ground black pepper

FENNEL SLAW

8 ounces fennel bulb

1 cup roughly chopped flat-leaf parsley

1 tablespoon balsamic vinegar or red wine vinegar

¼ cup fresh orange juice

1 tablespoon extra-virgin olive oil

1 teaspoon kosher salt

Freshly ground black pepper

Because of the "go big or go home" nature of cooking dry beans from scratch, this makes a big and filling pot of seriously hearty bean soup. It's ideal for those long wintery weeks in February; have a large batch on hand for brown-bag lunches and skip shuffling dreary, sleet-strewn workdays in search of lunch, or just enjoy some easy dinners at night. This soup is directly inspired by the mind-blowing cranberry bean soups you'll find during the winter at New York City's Superiority Burger; depending on the day, chef Brooks Headley may hand you a tiny cup of slow-simmered beans garnished with a petite ball of sticky rice or a layer of warm olive oil. You can easily steam up a little Steamed Sticky Rice (page 215) and drop some on top of each serving for that kind of business or make the refreshing fennel slaw for another nifty cool-hot entrée stew.

Sort the beans and discard any broken beans, pebbles, or random odd bits you'd rather not eat. Soak the beans overnight, or prepare them with a 1-hour speed soak (see note). Drain the soaking liquid and rinse the beans.

In a mortar and pestle, mash the garlic with a pinch of kosher salt into a rough paste, or if you prefer, mince the garlic.

Pour the olive oil into a 2-quart pot and heat over medium. When the oil shimmers, add the onion and celery. Fry for 5 minutes, or until the onion is tender and translucent. Add the garlic paste, bay leaves, and spices and fry for another minute. Add the beans, 6 cups of water, and the salt. Stir and increase the heat to high and bring to a rolling boil for 2 minutes, then reduce the heat to low. Partially cover and cook for 1½ hours, or until the beans are tender.

Add 1 cup of hot water and bring the beans to a boil again, then stir in the pasta. Cook for 6 minutes, or until the pasta is al dente (and not mushy). Turn off the heat and season with plenty of black pepper, and if desired a little more salt.

For the best flavor, I prefer to let the beans sit for 20 minutes to cool (scalding beans are never as tasty). During this cooling, reflective time, prepare the fennel slaw.

Remove the fronds and stems of the fennel. Dice the fennel into ½-inch pieces. In a mixing bowl, combine the fennel with the remaining slaw ingredients. Taste and adjust with more vinegar and salt if necessary. Chill the slaw until ready to serve.

Serve the soup warm with a scoop of fennel slaw on top. The soup will taste better the next day, and the fennel slaw will tenderize overnight, so you'll have a new and exciting soup-salad experience every day!

* SPEED SOAKING VERSUS OVERNIGHT

In an ideal world, we remember to sort, rinse, and soak our beans in cold water the night before. This way is best, but when perfection falls apart (as it will), the faster method is sort and rinse the beans, then boil in cold water for five minutes. Turn off the heat, cover, let stand for an hour. Drain and cook exactly like beans soaked overnight.

Tip

A little extra salt in a bean-and-pasta soup makes all the difference. Pasta needs assertively (read: *really*) salty water to taste its best, and the same goes for pasta cooked directly in soup. Beans love salted water too; it deepens flavors and textures. Don't be alarmed by the 3 teaspoons of kosher salt. As stated in the note on salt on page 13, I'm a stickler for Diamond kosher, which is a high-volume salt that's very forgiving when it comes to the potential to overly salt a dish. Using something other than Diamond kosher (sea salt or denser salt)? You may end up using only 2 teaspoons! Start with less in this recipe and taste the soup along the way, building up to the right level of salt.

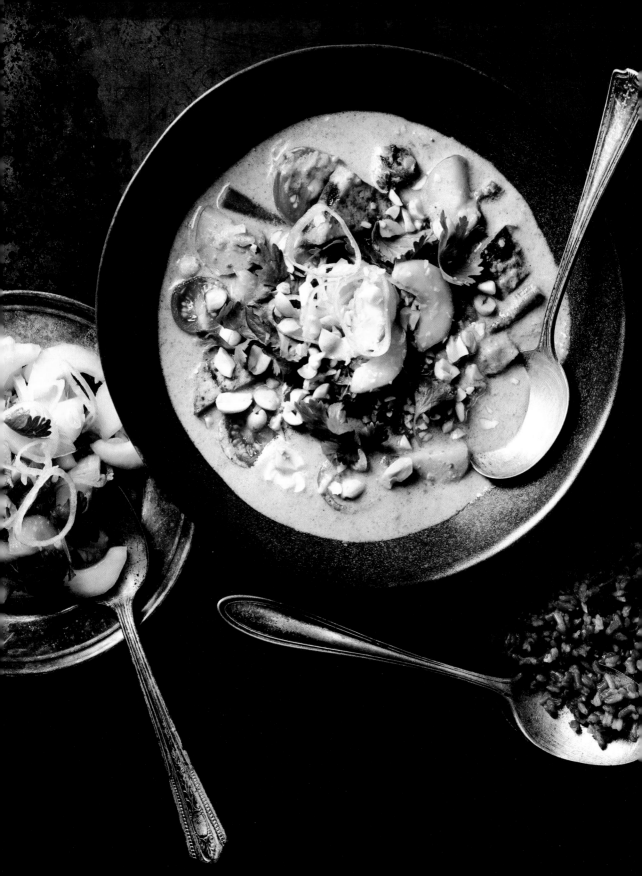

THAI PEANUT CURRY WITH QUICK CUCUMBER PICKLES

Serves 6

QUICK CUCUMBER PICKLES

2 garlic cloves

1 teaspoon kosher salt

3 tablespoons lime juice

1 pound hothouse (English or Persian) cucumbers, peeled, sliced in half and seeds removed, cut into ½-inch slices

1 medium red onion, peeled, quartered, and cut into ¼-inch slices

THAI PEANUT CURRY

2 tablespoons virgin coconut oil

2 garlic cloves, peeled

1-inch piece of ginger, peeled and sliced

1 teaspoon kosher salt, plus more for sprinkling

3 large shallots, peeled and thinly sliced

2 teaspoons garam masala powder

1 teaspoon Chinese 5-spice powder

½ teaspoon turmeric powder

1 to 2 Thai bird chiles, fresh or dried, minced, or ¼ to 1 teaspoon red pepper flakes

½ pound waxy potatoes, peeled and diced into ½-inch chunks

2 cups warm vegetable broth, divided

1 cup Thai full-fat coconut milk, stirred

½ cup chunky, all-natural peanut butter

1 tablespoon lime juice

2 teaspoons coconut sugar or organic dark brown sugar

6 slices of Sweet Lime Curry tofu (page 91), thinly sliced

1 cup cherry tomatoes, sliced in half

½ cup chopped roasted peanuts

1 cup roughly chopped cilantro, plus a little extra, for garnish

Lime wedges, for garnish

Continued

Massaman curry, the irresistible Thai peanut-coconut curry with intriguing Indian spices, is my favorite Thai curry, forever. But it is also surprisingly one of the easiest curries to make a tasty hack at home. A combination of Chinese 5-spice powder and Indian garam masala with just the right measure of spices is a stealthy shortcut for a richly fragrant curry, made even more exciting when paired with a refreshing quick cucumber pickles. Rice is always nice (again, Steamed Sticky Rice is calling, page 215), but for something different, serve with slabs of crusty baguette.

Prepare the pickle first, to give it some time to marinate and develop its optimal texture. In a mortar and pestle, pound the garlic with the salt into a paste, then scoop into a mixing bowl. Whisk in the lime juice, then fold in the cucumber and red onion slices. Cover and chill until ready to serve. Prior to starting the curry, start up your rice (according to the package directions or make the Steamed Sticky Rice).

In a 2-quart pot over medium heat, melt the coconut oil. With a mortar and pestle, pound the garlic, ginger, plus a big pinch of kosher salt into a chunky paste. Stir this into the coconut oil, add the shallots, and fry for 2 minutes. Stir in the garam masala, 5-spice powder, turmeric, and chiles and fry for 30 seconds. Add the potatoes and 1 cup of vegetable broth and coconut milk.

In a small mixing bowl, stir together the peanut butter and the remaining 1 cup of warm vegetable broth until

Continued

4 cups freshly made steaming-hot jasmine rice or Steamed Sticky Rice (page 215)

smooth. Use a rubber spatula to scoop the thinned-out peanut butter into the pot. Partially cover and bring the curry to a rapid simmer, then reduce the heat to low. Simmer, stirring occasionally, until the potatoes are very tender, about 20 to 25 minutes. Stir in the lime juice, coconut sugar, tofu, and cherry tomatoes. Continue to simmer another 5 minutes. Taste and adjust the seasonings with more salt, lime juice, and a pinch of sugar as desired, then remove from the heat. Stir in the chopped cilantro.

Ladle servings of curry into wide, generous serving bowls. Top with cucumber salad, chopped roasted peanuts, and a few cilantro leaves. Serve with lime wedges and hot rice. Spoon it up!

* Your friendly reminder for any recipe with a longer list of ingredients—use the principles of mise en place (page 4) to keep you calm and focused. For this recipe, I keep spices together into one small dish, put the chopped veggies that will be fried together in a bowl, and portion out the peanut butter into the same container for the broth. It's also helpful to put the things you'll go through first closer to the stove or burner, creating a curry-making assembly line.

VEGGIE NOODLE PHO WITH MICRO BAHN MI SALAD

Serves 4

VEGGIE NOODLE PHO

1 recipe Savory Sesame Tamari tofu (page 85), sliced into thin strips

1 (3-inch) piece ginger root, sliced in half lengthwise

2 large shallots (each about 2 inches long), unpeeled and sliced in half

8 cups vegetable broth

2 star anise

1 cinnamon stick

1 tablespoon coconut sugar or organic dark brown sugar

2 tablespoons lime juice

2 tablespoons tamari

4 cups spiraled vegetable noodles, such as butternut squash, zucchini, daikon, celeriac, sweet potato (see Two Notes About Noodles, below)

MICRO BAHN MI SALAD

¼ cup rice vinegar

1 tablespoon organic sugar

1 teaspoon kosher salt

1 cup peeled, julienned carrot

1 cup peeled, julienned daikon

1 cup torn cilantro leaves

½ cup coarsely chopped basil

½ cup coarsely chopped mint

2 large jalapeño peppers, sliced paper thin

2 scallions, white and tender green parts, thinly sliced

2 cups Naked Toasts (page 140)

There's a little Vietnamese joint in the Lower East Side, New York City, that serves a unique combo of a smallish bowl of vegan pho with half a tofu bahn mi; with just enough heady anise-scented noodle soup and just enough crusty, overfilled sandwich, it scratches each itch. This soup-salad combo offers yet another way to have your pho and bahn mi at the same time: hearty French bread croutons, tangy pickled vegetables, and steamy, gingery broth with crisp-soft veggie noodles. The croutons and lightly dressed salad are a sort of micro bahn mi sandwich, taken apart to garnish generous steaming bowls of vegetable noodle pho.

To lighten things up a bit, I've opted for veggie noodles in place of the usual rice or wheat noodles. And for the sake of time, while not authentic to the letter, speedy broth contains many of the automatic ingredients of traditional pho broth; don't skip out on the blackened onion, shallot, and ginger—it adds charred richness.

Make the tofu up to 2 days in advance. The croutons can be prepared up to a month in advance and re-toasted just before serving.

To make the pho broth, heat a cast-iron pan over high. Place the ginger and the shallots, cut-side down, on the hot, dry pan and grill until the cut sides are blackened, about 8 minutes.

In the meantime, set up a 3-quart stockpot and pour in the vegetable broth. Add the star anise, cinnamon, and sugar. Add the blackened vegetables, then bring the pot to gently boil over high heat. Reduce the heat to medium, partially cover, and actively simmer for 20 minutes.

Continued

Reduce the heat to low and use a long-handled wire skimmer (also called a spider skimmer) to remove the blackened veggies, star anise, and cinnamon stick. Stir in the lime juice and tamari. Taste the broth and adjust the seasoning as you like it, with a dash more of lime juice, tamari, or a pinch of coconut sugar or brown sugar. Add the veggie noodles, partially cover, and continue to simmer for another 5 to 8 minutes, or until the noodles are al dente, or your desired level of tenderness.

While the soup simmers, assemble the salad. In a mixing bowl, whisk together the vinegar, sugar, and salt. Fold in the carrot, daikon, cilantro, basil, mint, jalapeños, and scallions. Set aside to marinate until the soup is ready to serve.

To assemble, ladle the broth into wide, generously sized serving bowls. Use long-handled tongs to lift out a portion of veggie noodles into each bowl. Top each bowl with about ¾ cup of tofu strips. Add a handful of croutons, then top croutons with a generous portion of salad. Sprinkle any remaining marinade in the bowl over the salad and croutons. The pho is ready to eat!

variation

TWO NOTES ABOUT NOODLES

VEGGIE NOODLES

Spiralize at home or pick them up in the produce department; the kind of veggie noodle is entirely up to you. For a neutral pasta-like noodle, I love making celeriac noodles. Zucchini is tender, mild, and also blends in well. Butternut and sweet potato, while distinctively orange and sweet, are lovely with the harvest flavors of cinnamon and anise pho spices.

NO-VEGGIE NOODLES

Perhaps you're already eating *enough* salad and just want real noodles in your pho. Fair enough. Easy substitutes for this soup are Japanese soba and udon noodles, or use authentic Vietnamese pho noodles—narrow, flat, dried rice noodles that are cheap and plentiful in many Asian markets. I'd even recommend the new range of interesting rice ramen noodles on natural food store shelves, made with forbidden rice or Bhutan red or infused with turmeric or green tea. It's all great!

To use noodles for pho, cook according to the package directions, but cook only until al dente. Rinse cooked noodles with plenty of cold water to stop the cooking. Store in tightly sealed containers and cover with about an inch of water; noodles can stay this way for 2 days. When it's time to make pho, drain and rinse the noodles with warm water. Portion the noodles into serving bowls and ladle very hot broth over the noodles and prepare the rest of the soup as directed.

RED LENTIL KHICHDI WITH TWO CHUTNEYS

Serves 4 to 6

RED LENTIL KHICHDI

⅔ cup brown basmati rice

⅓ cup split red lentils

⅓ cup yellow split peas, mung dahl, or sprouted dried mung beans

1 to 2 cups hot water

2 teaspoons ground turmeric

½ teaspoon ground fenugreek

1½ teaspoons kosher salt

1 large white potato, scrubbed and diced

3 cups cauliflower florets

1 large carrot, scrubbed and diced small

6 ounces green beans, cut into 1-inch pieces

FRIED SPICE MIX

1 teaspoon black mustard seeds

2 tablespoons coconut oil or grape-seed oil

2 teaspoons cumin seeds

1 teaspoon fennel seeds

1 teaspoon nigella seeds (optional, but highly recommended)

1 tablespoon finely minced fresh ginger

1 hot green chile (jalapeno or serrano), minced

CILANTRO MINT COCONUT CHUTNEY

1 cup cilantro leaves, firmly packed

½ cup mint leaves, firmly packed

½ cup dried coconut

½ cup warm water

1 tablespoon lime juice

1 tablespoon coconut sugar

1 teaspoon kosher salt

Red Onion Quick Pickle (page 136)

Coconut Turmeric Lime chips (page 138)

Khichdi is Indian rice-and-lentils comfort food, a thick stew full of hearty vegetables and seasoned with lightly fried spices just before serving, often garnished with a simple chutney or pickle. I didn't grow up with khichdi, but I wish I had! It's soul food for winter days and the ideal one-pot meal.

This khichdi is much like a porridge (and not a rice pilaf), simmered for hours in the slow cooker to break down the lentils and rice into a creamy potage. Brown basmati rice and a nourishing mix of red lentils and mung beans (or other peas) create the basis of the dish. The addition of traditional mung dahl adds complexity (or try yellow split peas or get adventurous with sprouted dried mung beans). Chunky, sturdy vegetables (potatoes, cauliflower, green beans) stand up to the long simmer time and the bright chutney toppings— cilantro mint chutney and spicy crisp marinated onions (make both)—brighten the final dish. Beyond a light meal, it's amazing as a sugar-free, protein- and fiber-packed change from sweet oatmeal or sugary hot cereals.

Prepare the Red Onion Quick Pickle first and also, if desired, the cilantro chutney. These both can be made up to 2 days in advance. Keep chilled until ready to serve.

In a large mixing bowl, combine the rice, lentils, and peas. Rinse the mixture; add enough cool water to cover by 2 inches, swish the rice and lentils around, then drain off the water. Repeat 2 to 3 more times, or until the water no longer is cloudy and is almost clear. Cover everything with 2 inches of cold water once more and set aside to soak for at least 30 minutes (or cover and soak in the

Continued

fridge overnight). If cooking in a slow cooker, skip this presoaking step.

When you're ready to start cooking, drain the rice and transfer to a 2-quart cooking pot and add 5 cups of water, turmeric, fenugreek, and salt. Bring a rapid boil over high heat, stir, then reduce the heat to low and partially cover. Simmer for about 45 minutes to 1 hour, or until rice is very soft and red lentils look creamy.

Add the vegetables and another 2 cups of hot water, bring to a boil over high heat again, then reduce the heat to low. Simmer for 30 minutes until potatoes are tender. Turn off the heat and cover.

In a small, dry skillet over high heat, toast only the mustard seeds until they pop (cover with a lid to keep a hot mustard seed from flying into your eye). Dump the mustard seeds into the khichdi. Melt the coconut oil in the pan and the remaining spices, ginger, and chile and fry about 2 to 3 minutes until the ginger is soft. Pour this into the khichdi, using a silicone spatula to scrape every last drop of flavorful oil into the rice-lentil mixture. Stir and taste the khichdi, adding a little more salt to round out the flavor. Cover and prepare the chutney; the khichdi flavors will deepen the longer the flavors can meld.

To prepare the chutney, pulse everything in a food processor or blender until smooth. You'll likely need to push down the chutney occasionally with a rubber spatula to pulse the herbs, but it won't take very long. Scoop everything into a serving dish and chill any leftovers. I usually have enough chutney to go around for a few leftover servings of khichdi the next day.

Tip ────────────────────

SLOW COOKER COOKING

Slow cookers were made to make khichdi! The long, or overnight, simmering of rice and veggies with a quick flavoring finish at the end will put that underused slow cooker to work. In the cooler weather months, I regularly make a pot of this a week, changing up the veggies and occasionally the lentils and peas. It's rarely the exact same dish twice, and slow cookers make it ridiculously easy to make a fresh batch of khichdi a habit.

Rinse the rice, lentils, and peas. In a 2½-quart slow cooker, combine the rice, lentils, and peas with the turmeric, fenugreek, salt, and 4 cups of water. Simmer on high for 6 hours or low for 8 to 10 until rice is mushy and red lentils have fallen apart and have begun to look creamy.

Add the vegetables plus another 2 cups of water. Cover and increase the heat to high and simmer for 2 hours (or low for double the time). When the potatoes are tender, fry the spice mix and stir into the khichdi. Taste and adjust the seasoning and add more kosher salt, if desired. Serve hot with the chutneys!

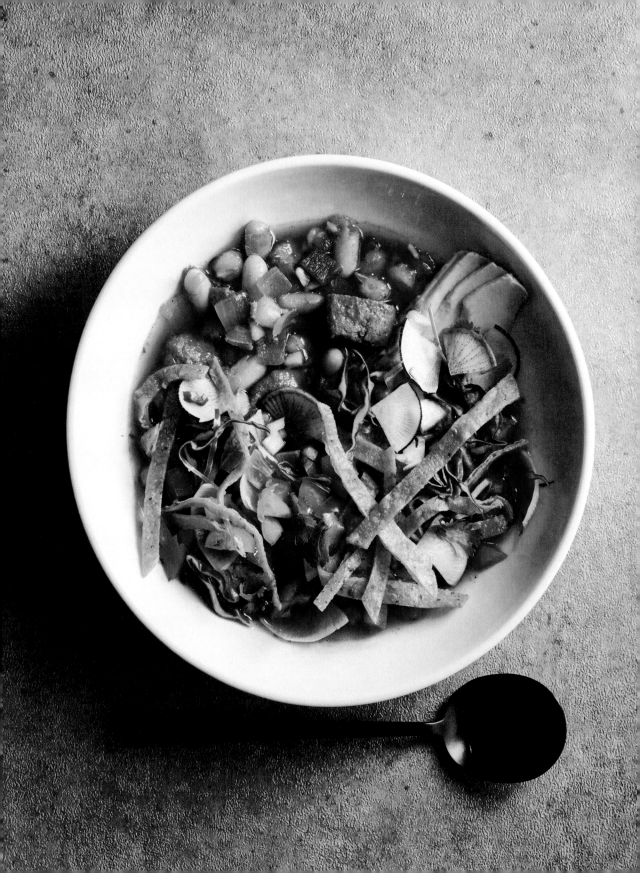

WHITE BEAN AND SEITAN GREEN POSOLE WITH AVOCADO RADISH SALAD

Serves 6

MARINATED SEITAN

8 ounces seitan, sliced into thin strips

2 tablespoons lime juice

2 garlic cloves, crushed

1 teaspoon kosher salt

2 tablespoons olive oil

POSOLE

¼ cup olive oil

1 large yellow onion, peeled, quartered, and cut into ¼-inch slices

4 garlic cloves, peeled and chopped

2 large poblano peppers, roasted and diced (see note below)

1 (14-ounce) can white beans (cannellini, navy, etc.), about 2 cups

1 (14-ounce) can hominy corn, rinsed very thoroughly

½ pound yellow waxy (such as Yukon Gold) potato, unpeeled and diced

2 teaspoons chili powder (such as New Mexican chili)

1 teaspoon ground cumin

1 teaspoon dried oregano

1 teaspoon kosher salt

4 cups vegetable broth

1 tablespoon lime juice

1 12-ounce bottle Mexican lager beer or 1⅓ cups vegetable broth

2 cups coarsely chopped spinach, kale, chard, or other similar greens

Posole, the family of Mexican soul food stews that share a common ingredient of hominy corn, is the beginning of my obsession with salad on soup. The brilliant contrast of steamy, brothy stew topped with cool, crunchy vegetables and tortilla strips shifted how I thought about soups forever, making me wonder why every soup didn't come loaded with cool, crunchy, crispy toppings. Even in meatless circles, there's room for so many different varieties. This subtle "green" spinach posole has a smoky edge from home-roasted poblano peppers, along with a creamy sweetness from white beans. And of course, you can shortcut the soup and use good-quality tortilla chips instead of making strips out of tortillas.

Prepare the seitan if using (it can be made up to a week in advance). In a glass container, whisk together the seitan marinade ingredients. Add the sliced seitan, cover, shake to coat with the marinade, and marinate for up to 2 days in the fridge. If serving with Crumbly, Salty Almond Cheese, prepare that 2 days (up to a month) in advance.

Start the soup: In a 2-quart soup pot over medium heat, heat the oil until it shimmers and stir in the onion and garlic. Fry until the onion is soft and transparent, about 3 minutes, then stir in the diced poblano peppers. Add the marinated seitan and fry for 4 minutes, or until the strips are just starting to get brown on the edges.

Continued

Continued

AVOCADO RADISH SALAD

4 red globe radishes, scrubbed and thinly diced, about 1 cup

1 cup shredded red cabbage

½ cup white or red onion, finely diced

½ cup roughly chopped cilantro

1 large tomato, diced

2 tablespoons lime juice

1 teaspoon kosher salt

1 ripe Haas avocado, pit removed and diced

TOPPINGS

4 corn or whole-wheat flour tortillas

1 tablespoon olive oil

1 cup crumbled Crumbly, Salty Almond Cheese (page 113—nice but not necessary)

Additional cilantro sprigs

Add the beans, hominy, potato, chili powder, cumin, oregano, salt, broth, lime juice, and beer. Increase the heat to medium-high and bring the soup to a rapid simmer for 5 minutes, then reduce the heat to low and partially cover. Simmer the soup for another 25 to 35 minutes, or until the hominy and potato are very tender. Stir in the greens and simmer for another 2 minutes to wilt the greens. Turn off the heat and keep covered until it's time to serve.

Preheat the oven to 350°F and brush the corn tortillas on both sides with oil. Cut into 1-inch-wide strips. Toast the tortillas for 4 to 6 minutes until crisp and browned. Promptly remove from the oven to prevent burning.

While the soup is simmering, in a large mixing bowl, toss together all the salad ingredients except the avocado. Cover and allow it to marinate until it's serving time. Just before serving, fold in the diced avocado.

Ladle the soup into wide, generous serving bowls. Top with tortilla strips and a big scoop of salad, and garnish with cilantro sprigs and a few crumbles of almond cheese, if using, and serve with lime wedges.

* About the seitan: I've been making a quick, steamed seitan for years, but if I can find it, I use a seasoned, off-the-shelf seitan for this dish. Blackbird and Upton's are two of my favorite brands available in pre-seasoned, ready-to-use 8-ounce packages.

ROASTING POBLANOS

Roast a poblano (or any chile pepper) by placing the pepper directly on a gas burner on high flame. Use long-handled tongs to rotate the pepper until all the sides are charred and the pepper looks slightly collapsed. Transfer to a bowl, cover with a plate, and set aside to cool for 5 minutes. When it is cool enough to handle, peel (the pepper will self-steam and loosen up the skin) and discard the charred skin, seeds, and stems.

METRIC CONVERSION CHART

The recipes in this book have not been tested with metric measurements, so some variations might occur. Remember that the weight of dry ingredients varies according to the volume or density factor; 1 cup of flour weighs far less than 1 cup of sugar, and 1 tablespoon doesn't necessarily hold 3 teaspoons.

GENERAL FORMULA FOR METRIC CONVERSION

Ounces to grams	multiply ounces by 28.35
Grams to ounces	multiply grams by 0.035
Pounds to grams	multiply pounds by 453.5
Pounds to kilograms	multiply pounds by 0.45
Cups to liters	multiply cups by 0.24
Fahrenheit to Celsius	subtract 32 from Fahrenheit temperature, multiply by 5, divide by 9
Celsius to Fahrenheit	multiply Celsius temperature by 9, divide by 5, add 32

VOLUME (LIQUID) MEASUREMENTS

1 teaspoon	= ⅙ fluid ounce	= 5 milliliters
1 tablespoon	= ½ fluid ounce	= 15 milliliters
2 tablespoons	= 1 fluid ounce	= 30 milliliters
¼ cup	= 2 fluid ounces	= 60 milliliters
⅓ cup	= 2⅔ fluid ounces	= 79 milliliters
½ cup	= 4 fluid ounces	= 118 milliliters
1 cup or ½ pint	= 8 fluid ounces	= 250 milliliters
2 cups or 1 pint	= 16 fluid ounces	= 500 milliliters
4 cups or 1 quart	= 32 fluid ounces	= 1,000 milliliters
1 gallon	= 4 liters	

WEIGHT (MASS) MEASUREMENTS

1 ounce	= 30 grams	
2 ounces	= 55 grams	
3 ounces	= 85 grams	
4 ounces	= ¼ pound	= 125 grams
8 ounces	= ½ pound	= 240 grams
12 ounces	= ¾ pound	= 375 grams
16 ounces	= 1 pound	= 454 grams

OVEN TEMPERATURE EQUIVALENTS, FAHRENHEIT (F) AND CELSIUS (C)

100°F	= 38°C
200°F	= 95°C
250°F	= 120°C
300°F	= 150°C
350°F	= 180°C
400°F	= 205°C
450°F	= 230°C

VOLUME (DRY) MEASUREMENTS

¼ teaspoon	= 1 milliliter
½ teaspoon	= 2 milliliters
¾ teaspoon	= 4 milliliters
1 teaspoon	= 5 milliliters
1 tablespoon	= 15 milliliters
¼ cup	= 59 milliliters
⅓ cup	= 79 milliliters
½ cup	= 118 milliliters
⅔ cup	= 158 milliliters
¾ cup	= 177 milliliters
1 cup	= 225 milliliters
4 cups or 1 quart	= 1 liter
½ gallon	= 2 liters
1 gallon	= 4 liters

LINEAR MEASUREMENTS

½ inch	= 1¼ cm
1 inch	= 2½ cm
6 inches	= 15 cm
8 inches	= 20 cm
10 inches	= 25 cm
12 inches	= 30 cm
20 inches	= 50 cm

ACKNOWLEDGMENTS

Cookbooks require a tremendous amount of effort. The following amazing humans were essential to the creation of this work.

My incredibly patient editor, Renee Sedilar, project editor Michael Clark, Sara and Chris Ensey, and the staff at Perseus.

My agent, Marc Gerald.

Vanessa Rees, my brilliant food photographer, and the studio crew—Mélanie Duault, Bernadette Mira, Tala Soubra—for long days of hard work, good times, and great salad lunches.

Marisa Ford, brilliant vegan chef in her own right, who helped me test recipes, worked tirelessly preparing countless things for the photo shoot, and for her gift of vegan pastries and upbeat spirit, which kept us all going.

Liz Stretch, wise teacher and student of food and clay, creator of many of the rustically sublime platters, dishes, and bowls seen in these photos. Visit her work on Instagram at @stretchceramics.

Derrick Hachey, my partner in adventure and endless batches of hot sauce.

John Stavropolous, my best friend. And the support and inspiration near and afar from Russell Heiman, Jess and James and Rachel and John at Woodstock Farm Sanctuary, Brooks Headley for mind-blowing vegetable inspo at Superiority Burger, Erica and Sarah and the Orchard Grocery team.

And a special thanks to the following for lending their cooking efforts toward testing these recipes: Lisa Dawn Angerame, Melanie Chang, Michelle Fleming, Carla Kelly, Chris Kim, Emily Lavieri-Scull, Chris Moultrie, Todd Schmiedlin, and Jackie Smith.

INDEX

Note: Page references in *italics* indicate photographs.

A

Aburaage, Marinated Pan-Fried, 80

Almond(s)
Cheese, Crumbly, Salty, *112*, 113–115
Crunch, Crispy, Cheesy, *116*, 117
Potato Leek Soup with Broccoli Gremolata, 247–249, *248*
and Red Pepper Romesco Dressing, 52
and Roasted Chickpeas, Mustard Greens Tabbouleh with, 222–224, *223*
Sweet, Salty, Nutty Gomasio, 148

Apple(s)
The Big Crunchy Autumn Vibes Salad, *158*, 159
The Bold and Bountiful Winter Salad, 160, *161*
Chickpea Pickle Collard Wraps, 170–172, *171*
Green Again Soup with Tahini Miso Slaw, *252*, 253
storing, 20
Walnut Salad, Creamy Cauliflower Soup with, 254–256, *255*

Arugula
The Bright and Spicy Spring Asparagus Salad, 151–152, *153*
The Juicy Grilled Summer Days Peach Salad, *154*, 155–156
Pepita Greenest Goddess Dressing, 51
Pizza Panzanella with Beet Prosciutto, *234*, 235–236
Roasted Ratatouille Salad with Romesco Dressing, 201–203, *202*

Asparagus Salad, The Bright and Spicy Spring, 151–152, *153*

Avocado(s)
All-Day Breakfast Nacho Salad Bowl, 192–194, *193*
and Black Bean Salad on Cornbread Toast, 243–244, *245*
Collard Salad, Ethiopian Red Lentils with Butternut and, 257–259, *258*
Korean Shiitake Bacon Salad Rice Bowl, 219–221, *220*
Peanut Brown Rice Crunch Bowl, *210*, 211
Protein-Packed Salad for Breakfast, *190*, 191

Radish Salad, White Bean and Seitan Green Posole with, *272*, 273–274

B

Bacon
Korean Shiitake, Salad Rice Bowl, 219–221, *220*
Maple Mushroom, 125–126
Roasted Cabbage Steak with Peanut Sauce and Fried Shallots, 186–187
Root, 127–128, *129*
Root, Charred Broccoli, and Potato Salad, 229–230

Balsamic
Dijon Vinaigrette, 71
Orange Vinaigrette, The Best, 72
White, Dressing, 69

Basil
Crunchy Eggplant Parm Salad, *206*, 207–208
The Juicy Grilled Summer Days Peach Salad, *154*, 155–156
Pesto Croutons, 140
Pizza Panzanella with Beet Prosciutto, *234*, 235–236

Roasted Ratatouille Salad
with Romesco Dressing,
201–203, *202*
Roasted Tomato Chickpea
Pasta Salad, 231–232,
233
Thai, Spaghetti Squash with
Curry Tofu, 181–182, *183*
Bean(s). *See also* Chickpea(s);
Green Beans
Black, and Avocado Salad
on Cornbread Toast,
243–244, *245*
The Bright and Spicy Spring
Asparagus Salad,
151–152, *153*
Cranberry, and Pasta Stew
with Fennel Slaw,
262–263
dried, for recipes, 11
Homemade, 106–107
Orange Collard Greens, Corn,
and Black-Eyed Peas,
173–175, *174*
White, and Seitan Green
Posole with Avocado
Radish Salad, *272,*
273–274
White, Salt-and-Pepper Fried,
102
Beet Prosciutto, 131–133, *132*
Beet Prosciutto, Pizza Panzanella
with, *234,* 235–236
Berries, storing, 20
Black-Eyed Peas, Collard
Greens, and Corn,
Orange, 173–175, *174*
Black peppercorns, cracking, 47
Black sesame seeds, about, 12
Blenders, 10
Bok choy
Green Again Soup with Tahini
Miso Slaw, *252, 253*
Breads. *See also* Croutons
Avocado and Black Bean
Salad on Cornbread
Toast, 243–244, *245*

Greek Golden Fava Salad
Pita, *240,* 241–242
Naked Toasts, 140
Vegan Cornbread Loaf, 146,
147
Zucchini and Chickpea
Fattoush Salad, 237–238,
239
Broccoli
Charred, Potato, and Root
Bacon Salad, 229–230
Gremolata, Potato Leek Soup
with, 247–249, *248*
and Tofu Salad, General Tso's,
184, 185
Brussels sprouts
Green Again Soup with Tahini
Miso Slaw, *252,* 253
Buffalo Hot Sauce Marinade, 84
Buffalo Tofu, Butternut Squash,
and Kale Bowl, 176, *177*
Buffalo Tomato Soup with Kale
Caesar Salad, 250, *251*
Bulgur wheat
Mustard Greens Tabbouleh
with Almonds and
Roasted Chickpeas,
222–224, *223*

C

Cabbage
All-Day Breakfast Nacho Salad
Bowl, 192–194, *193*
Blackened Tempeh Reuben
Salad, *178,* 179
The Bold and Bountiful Winter
Salad, 160, *161*
Buffalo Tofu, Butternut
Squash, and Kale Bowl,
176, *177*
Peking-Roasted Tofu Noodle
Salad, *216,* 217–218
Sriracha Tofu Lettuce Wraps
with Peanut Dressing,
168, 169

Steak, Roasted, with Peanut
Sauce and Fried Shallots,
186–187
Thai Basil Spaghetti Squash
with Curry Tofu, 181–182,
183
Caesar Dressings
Hemp Seed, *30,* 31
Sun and Sea Sunflower, 39
Caesar Salads
Classic Romaine, 164
Forever Kale, with Cheesy,
Crispy Croutons, *162,*
163–164
Kale, Buffalo Tomato Soup
with, 250, *251*
Restaurant-Style Entrée, 164
Caesar Walnuts, *122,* 123
Canned pantry staples, 11
Carrot(s)
Baby, Ginger Soup with
Sesame Slaw, 260–261
Ginger Dressing, 58
Pastrami, 130
Root Bacon, 127–128, *129*
Thai Basil Spaghetti Squash
with Curry Tofu, 181–182,
183
Veggie Noodle Pho with Micro
Bahn Mi Salad, 267–268
Cashew(s)
Cucumber Dill Dressing,
48–49
Lemon Pepper Dressing, Oil-
Free, 46–47
Peanut Avocado Brown Rice
Crunch Bowl, 210, *211*
Spicy Cucumber and Curry
Tofu Salad with Sticky
Rice, 212–215, *213*
Thai Basil Spaghetti Squash
with Curry Tofu, 181–182,
183
unroasted raw pieces, about, 28
Cauliflower
Green Again Soup with Tahini
Miso Slaw, *252,* 253

Korean Shiitake Bacon Salad
Rice Bowl, 219–221, *220*
Red Lentil Khichdi with Two
Chutneys, 269–271
Soup, Creamy, with Apple
Walnut Salad, 254–256,
255
steaks, preparing, 200
Celery
The Big Crunchy Autumn
Vibes Salad, *158,* 159
Chickpea Pickle Collard
Wraps, 170–172, *171*
Creamy Cauliflower Soup
with Apple Walnut Salad,
254–256, *255*
Chard
All-Day Breakfast Nacho
Salad Bowl, 192–194,
193
The Bright and Spicy Spring
Asparagus Salad,
151–152, *153*
Roasted Tomato Chickpea
Pasta Salad, 231–232,
233
White Bean and Seitan Green
Posole with Avocado
Radish Salad, *272,*
273–274
Cheese
All-Day Breakfast Nacho
Salad Bowl, 192–194,
193
Almond, Crumbly, Salty, *112,*
113–115
Chic Melts, *171,* 172
Chia (seeds)
adding to dressing, 47
Croutons, No-Oil, 141
Chickpea(s)
Pickle Collard Wraps,
170–172, *171*
Roasted, and Almonds,
Mustard Greens
Tabbouleh with, 222–224,
223

Roasted Lemon Pepper,
100–101
Roasted Niçoise Salad, 188,
189
Roasted Tomato Pasta Salad,
231–232, *233*
White Sweet Potato Salad
with Spinach Zhug
Dressing, 198–200, *199*
and Zucchini Fattoush Salad,
237–238, *239*
Chile(s)
Aji Amarillo Dressing, 225
Green Curry Paste, 196
Lime Marinade, Peruvian, 87
poblano, roasting directions,
274
Spinach Zhug Dressing,
198–200, *199*
Thai bird, about, 12
White Bean and Seitan Green
Posole with Avocado
Radish Salad, *272,*
273–274
Chipotle Bacon Coconut Chips,
138
Chutney, Cilantro Mint Coconut,
269–271
Cilantro
Green Again Soup with Tahini
Miso Slaw, *252,* 253
Green Curry Paste, 196
Kabocha and Black Rice
Salad, 195–196, *197*
Mint Coconut Chutney,
269–271
Peruvian Potato and Red
Quinoa Salad, 225–227,
226
Roasted Cabbage Steak with
Peanut Sauce and Fried
Shallots, 186–187
Spinach Zhug Dressing,
198–200, *199*
Sriracha Ranch Dressing,
40, *41*
Thai Basil Spaghetti Squash

with Curry Tofu, 181–182,
183
Thai Peanut Curry with Quick
Cucumber Pickles, *264,*
265–266
Veggie Noodle Pho with Micro
Bahn Mi Salad, 267–268
Citrus juice, buying, 28
Coconut
Chips, Savory, 3 Ways, 138
Cilantro Mint Chutney,
269–271
Peanut Dressing, Sultry, 54
Collard(s)
Avocado Salad, Ethiopian Red
Lentils with Butternut and,
257–259, *258*
Greens, Corn, and Black-Eyed
Peas, Orange, 173–175,
174
Protein-Packed Salad for
Breakfast, *190,* 191
Wraps, Chickpea Pickle,
170–172, *171*
Condiments, for recipes, 12
Coriander Bird Marinade, Golden,
93
Corn
Collard Greens, and Black-
Eyed Peas, Orange,
173–175, *174*
Pan-Roasted Chile, 134
Peruvian Potato and Red
Quinoa Salad, 225–227,
226
Cornbread
Crunch, Herbed, *144,* 145
Loaf, Vegan, 146, *147*
Toast, Avocado and Black
Bean Salad on, 243–244,
245
Cranberries
The Big Crunchy Autumn
Vibes Salad, *158,* 159
Orange Collard Greens, Corn,
and Black-Eyed Peas,
173–175, *174*

Croutons
Cheesy, Crispy, 142, *143*
Cheesy, Crispy, Forever
Kale Caesar with, *162,*
163–164
Herbed Cornbread Crunch,
144, 145
No-Oil Chia, 141
Seedy Garlic Bread, 139–140
Simple, 140
storing, 21
Cucumber(s)
and Curry Tofu Salad,
Spicy, with Sticky Rice,
212–215, *213*
Dill Dressing, 48–49
Greek Golden Fava Salad
Pita, *240,* 241–242
Lazy Seitan Gyro Spinach
Salad, 204–205, *206*
Mustard Greens Tabbouleh
with Almonds and
Roasted Chickpeas,
222–224, *223*
Peanut Avocado Brown Rice
Crunch Bowl, *210,* 211
Peking-Roasted Tofu Noodle
Salad, *216,* 217–218
Pickles, Quick, *264,* 265–266
Roasted Cabbage Steak with
Peanut Sauce and Fried
Shallots, 186–187
Sriracha Ranch Salad Party,
165–166, *167*
Thai Basil Spaghetti Squash
with Curry Tofu, 181–182,
183
Curry, Thai Peanut, with Quick
Cucumber Pickles, *264,*
265–266
Curry Lime Marinade, Sweet, 91
Curry Paste, Green, 196
Curry Tofu, Thai Basil Spaghetti
Squash with, 181–182,
183

D

Dill Cucumber Dressing, 48–49
Dressings. *See also* Vinaigrettes
Aji Amarillo, 225
Carrot Ginger, 58
Cashew Lemon Pepper, Oil-
Free, 46–47
creamy, nondairy milks for, 29
creamy, nuts and seeds for, 28
Creamy Italian Hemp, 33
Cucumber Dill, 48–49
Deep Dark Sesame, 55
essential ingredients for, 27
Ginger Garlic Fire, 57
Gojuchang, 221
Hemp Seed Caesar, *30,* 31
Hemp Seed Tarragon Dijon,
32
Hollyhock, 61
Horseradish Hemp, 34
layering of, 26
New Catalina, 62, *63*
Pepita Greenest Goddess, 51
Red Pepper and Almond
Romesco, 52
Roasted Pico de Gallo, 59
Salted Lemon Pepper, 47
Spinach Zhug, 198–200, *199*
Sriracha Cilantro Ranch, 40,
41
storing, 21
Sultry Peanut Coconut, 54
Sun and Sea Sunflower
Caesar, 39
Sun-Dried Tomato, 60
Sunflower Ranch, *36,* 37–38,
49
Tahini, 43
Tahini French, 45
tossing, with salad ingredients,
27–28
Turmeric Tahini Miso Sauce,
44
Wasabi Miso Lime, 56
White Balsamic, 69

E

Eggplant
Fries, Crunchy, *206,* 207–208
Parm Salad, Crunchy, *206,*
207–208
Roasted Ratatouille Salad
with Romesco Dressing,
201–203, *202*
Ethiopian Red Lentils with
Butternut and Avocado
Collard Salad, 257–259,
258

F

Fattoush Salad, Zucchini and
Chickpea, 237–238, *239*
Fennel
The Bold and Bountiful Winter
Salad, 160, *161*
Roasted Ratatouille Salad
with Romesco Dressing,
201–203, *202*
Slaw, Cranberry Bean
and Pasta Stew with,
262–263
Fiddleheads, adding to salad, 152
French Dressing, Tahini, 45
Fruits. *See also specific fruits*
storing, 20

G

Garlic
Bread Croutons, Seedy,
139–140
Ginger Fire Dressing, 57
Oregano Lemon Vinaigrette,
69
storing, 20
Ginger
Baby Carrot Soup with
Sesame Slaw, 260–261

Carrot Dressing, 58
Garlic Fire Dressing, 57
Gluten-free recipes, ingredient
    swaps for, 21
Gojuchang, about, 12
Gojuchang Dressing, 221
Gomasio, Sweet, Salty, Nutty,
    148
Grains. *See also* Quinoa; Rice
    cooked, storing, 21
    Mustard Greens Tabbouleh
        with Almonds and
        Roasted Chickpeas,
        222–224, *223*
    substituting, in Tabbouleh, 224
Greek Golden Fava Salad Pita,
    240, 241–242
Green Beans
    Roasted Niçoise Salad, 188,
        189
    Spicy Cucumber and Curry
        Tofu Salad with Sticky
        Rice, 212–215, *213*
Green Curry Paste, 196
Greens. *See also specific greens*
    choosing, 5
    Crunchy Eggplant Parm Salad,
        206, 207–208
    Mustard, Tabbouleh with
        Almonds and Roasted
        Chickpeas, 222–224,
        223
    Peanut Avocado Brown Rice
        Crunch Bowl, *210,* 211
    Protein-Packed Salad for
        Breakfast, *190,* 191
    Roasted Niçoise Salad, 188,
        189
    soaking, 5
    storing, 20
    washing and drying, 5–6
    White Sweet Potato Salad
        with Spinach Zhug
        Dressing, 198–200, *199*

H

Hazelnuts, Bacon Crunch, 121
Hemp Seed(s)
    about, 29
    Caesar Dressing, *30,* 31
    Creamy Italian Hemp
        Dressing, 33
    Horseradish Hemp Dressing, 34
    Seedy Garlic Bread Croutons,
        139–140
    Tarragon Dijon Dressing, 32
Herbs. *See also specific herbs*
    dried, for recipes, 11
    Herbed Cornbread Crunch,
        144, 145
    No-Oil Chia Croutons, 141
    Pepita Greenest Goddess
        Dressing, 51
    storing, 20
    Sunflower Ranch Dressing,
        36, 37–38, *49*
Hollyhock Dressing, 61
Horseradish Hemp Dressing, 34
Hot Sauce Buffalo Marinade, 84

I

Immersion blenders, 10
Italian Hemp Dressing, Creamy,
    33

J

Japanese mandoline, 9–10

K

Kale
    The Big Crunchy Autumn
        Vibes Salad, *158,* 159
    Blackened Tempeh Reuben
        Salad, *178,* 179

The Bold and Bountiful Winter
    Salad, 160, *161*
Buffalo Tofu, and Butternut
    Squash Bowl, 176, *177*
Caesar, Forever, with Cheesy,
    Crispy Croutons, *162,*
    163–164
Caesar Salad, Buffalo Tomato
    Soup with, 250, *251*
Green Again Soup with Tahini
    Miso Slaw, *252,* 253
Protein-Packed Salad for
    Breakfast, *190,* 191
Restaurant-Style Entrée
    Caesar, 164
White Bean and Seitan Green
    Posole with Avocado
    Radish Salad, *272,*
    273–274
Khichdi, Red Lentil, with Two
    Chutneys, 269–271
Kitchen tools, 7–10
Knives, 7–8
Korean BBQ Marinade, 86
Korean BBQ Shiitakes, 86
Korean red pepper powder,
    about, 12
Korean Shiitake Bacon Salad
    Rice Bowl, 219–221, *220*

L

Leeks, cleaning, 249
Legumes. *See also* Bean(s);
    Lentil(s)
    dried, for recipes, 11
Lemon(s)
    Dijon Marinade, *88,* 89
    juice, buying, 28
    Maple Vinaigrette, Bright &
        Tangy, 68
    Oregano Garlic Vinaigrette, 69
    Pepper Cashew Dressing, Oil-
        Free, 46–47
    Pepper Chickpeas, Roasted,
        100–101

Salted, 64–65
Salted, Pepper Dressing, 47
Lentil(s)
Dressed, 104
Protein-Packed Salad for
Breakfast, *190,* 191
for recipes, 11
Red, Ethiopian, with Butternut
and Avocado Collard
Salad, 257–259, *258*
Red, Khichdi with Two
Chutneys, 269–271
Roasted Ratatouille Salad
with Romesco Dressing,
201–203, *202*
Lettuce
All-Day Breakfast Nacho
Salad Bowl, 192–194,
193
The Big Crunchy Autumn
Vibes Salad, *158,* 159
Classic Romaine Caesar, 164
Greek Golden Fava Salad
Pita, *240,* 241–242
The Juicy Grilled Summer
Days Peach Salad, *154,*
155–156
Roasted Niçoise Salad, 188,
189
Sriracha Ranch Salad Party,
165–166, *167*
Wraps, Sriracha Tofu, with
Peanut Dressing, *168,*
169
Zucchini and Chickpea
Fattoush Salad, 237–238,
239
Lime
-and-Salt Shallots, Crispy, 135
Chile Marinade, Peruvian, 87
Curry Marinade, Sweet, 91
juice, buying, 28
Turmeric Coconut Chips, 138
Wasabi Miso Dressing, 56

M

Mandoline, 9–10
Maple (syrup)
Almost Like Bacon Marinade,
94
Bacon Crunch Nuts and
Seeds, 120–121
Lemon Vinaigrette, Bright &
Tangy, 68
Mushroom Bacon, 125–126
Mustard Shallot Vinaigrette,
70
Marinades
Golden Coriander Bird, 93
Hot Sauce Buffalo, 84
Korean BBQ, 86
Lemon Dijon, *88,* 89
Maple Almost Like Bacon, 94
Peruvian Chile Lime, 87
Savory Sesame Tamari, 85
Sriracha Orange, 90
storing, 21
Sweet Lime Curry, 91
Tahini Miso, 92
Mason jars, 10
Mayo, Tahini, 43
Microgreens, growing, 14–16
Mint
Cilantro Coconut Chutney,
269–271
Mustard Greens Tabbouleh
with Almonds and
Roasted Chickpeas,
222–224, *223*
Thai Basil Spaghetti Squash
with Curry Tofu, 181–182,
183
Veggie Noodle Pho with Micro
Bahn Mi Salad, 267–268
Miso
Tahini Marinade, 92
Tahini Slaw, Green Again
Soup with, *252,* 253
Turmeric Tahini Sauce, 44
Wasabi Lime Dressing, 56
Mixing bowls, 9

Mushroom(s)
Korean BBQ Shiitakes, 86
Maple Bacon, 125–126
Mustard
Balsamic Dijon Vinaigrette, 71
Ginger Garlic Fire Dressing,
57
Hemp Seed Tarragon Dijon
Dressing, 32
Lemon Dijon Marinade, *88,* 89
Maple Shallot Vinaigrette, 70
Mustard Greens
Protein-Packed Salad for
Breakfast, *190,* 191
Tabbouleh with Almonds and
Roasted Chickpeas,
222–224, *223*

N

Noodle(s). *See also* Veggie
Noodle(s)
kelp, about, 168
Kelp, Peking Tofu, 218
Peking-Roasted Tofu Salad,
216, 217–218
for pho, preparing, 268
Roasted Cabbage Steak with
Peanut Sauce and Fried
Shallots, 186–187
soba, about, 12
Sriracha Tofu Lettuce Wraps
with Peanut Dressing,
168, 169
Nutritional yeast
about, 12
Cheesy, Crispy Croutons, 142,
143
Crispy, Cheesy Almond
Crunch, *116,* 117
Crunchy Eggplant Parm Salad,
206, 207–208
Hollyhock Dressing, 61
Nut-Free, Soy-Free Cheesy
Sunflower Crunch, 118,
119

Toasted Sun and Pepita Parm,
110
Nut(s). *See also specific nuts*
-based toppings, storing,
21
for creamy dairy-free
dressings, 28
-free recipes, ingredient
swaps for, 21
for recipes, 11
and Seeds, Bacon Crunch,
120–121

O

Oils, 11
Olives
Greek Golden Fava Salad
Pita, *240,* 241–242
Lazy Seitan Gyro Spinach
Salad, 204–205, *206*
Peruvian Potato and Red
Quinoa Salad, 225–227,
226
Pizza Panzanella with Beet
Prosciutto, *234,* 235–236
Roasted Niçoise Salad, 188,
189
Onion(s)
Red, Quick Pickle, 136
storing, 20
Orange
Balsamic Vinaigrette, The
Best, 72
Sriracha Marinade, 90
Oregano Garlic Lemon
Vinaigrette, 69

P

Panzanella, Pizza, with Beet
Prosciutto, *234,* 235–236
Parsley
Baby Carrot Ginger Soup with
Sesame Slaw, 260–261

Green Again Soup with Tahini
Miso Slaw, *252, 253*
Mustard Greens Tabbouleh
with Almonds and
Roasted Chickpeas,
222–224, *223*
Potato Leek Soup with
Broccoli Gremolata,
247–249, *248*
Spinach Zhug Dressing,
198–200, *199*
Zucchini and Chickpea
Fattoush Salad, 237–238,
239
Parsnips
Creamy Cauliflower Soup
with Apple Walnut Salad,
254–256, *255*
Root Bacon, 127–128, *129*
Pasta
cooked, storing, 21
and Cranberry Bean Stew with
Fennel Slaw, 262–263
Roasted Tomato Chickpea
Salad, 231–232, *233*
Pastrami, Tempeh, Whole-Loaf
Blackened, *96,* 97–98
Pastrami Carrots, 130
Peach Salad, The Juicy Grilled
Summer Days, *154,*
155–156
Peanut butter
Sultry Peanut Coconut
Dressing, 54
Thai Peanut Curry with Quick
Cucumber Pickles, *264,*
265–266
Peanut(s)
Avocado Brown Rice Crunch
Bowl, *210,* 211
General Tso's Tofu and
Broccoli Salad, *184,* 185
Peruvian Potato and Red
Quinoa Salad, 225–227,
226
7-Spice, 111
Spicy Cucumber and Curry

Tofu Salad with Sticky
Rice, 212–215, *213*
Thai Peanut Curry with Quick
Cucumber Pickles, *264,*
265–266
Pears
The Big Crunchy Autumn
Vibes Salad, *158,* 159
The Bold and Bountiful Winter
Salad, 160, *161*
Peas
Black-Eyed, Collard Greens,
and Corn, Orange,
173–175, *174*
The Bright and Spicy Spring
Asparagus Salad,
151–152, *153*
Sriracha Tofu Lettuce Wraps
with Peanut Dressing,
168, 169
Peas, split. *See* Split peas
Pecans
Bacon Crunch, 121
Sweet and Salty, 121
Pepita(s)
Bacon Crunch Nuts and
Seeds, 120–121
Greenest Goddess Dressing,
51
Toasted Sun and Pepita Parm,
110
Peppercorns, cracking, 47
Pepper(s). *See also* Chile(s)
Red, and Almond Romesco
Dressing, 52
red, roasting directions,
53
Roasted Ratatouille Salad
with Romesco Dressing,
201–203, *202*
Peruvian Chile Lime Marinade,
87
Peruvian Potato and Red Quinoa
Salad, 225–227, *226*
Pesto, Basil, Croutons, 140
Pho, Veggie Noodle, with Micro
Bahn Mi Salad, 267–268

Pickle(s)
    Chickpea Collard Wraps,
        170–172, *171*
    Quick, Red Onion, 136
    Quick Cucumber, *264,*
        265–266
Pico de Gallo, Roasted, Dressing,
    59
Pizza, Salad, 166
Pomegranate molasses, about,
    238
Pomegranate Vinaigrette, 69
Posole, White Bean and Seitan
    Green, with Avocado
    Radish Salad, *272,*
    273–274
Potato(es). *See also* Sweet
    Potato(es)
    All-Day Breakfast Nacho
        Salad Bowl, 192–194,
        193
    The Bold and Bountiful Winter
        Salad, 160, *161*
    Charred Broccoli, and Root
        Bacon Salad, 229–230
    Leek Soup with Broccoli
        Gremolata, 247–249, *248*
    and Red Quinoa Salad,
        Peruvian, 225–227, *226*
    Roasted Niçoise Salad, 188,
        189
    storing, 20
    Thai Peanut Curry with Quick
        Cucumber Pickles, *264,*
        265–266
Prosciutto, Beet, 131–133, *132*
Prosciutto, Beet, Pizza Panzanella
    with, *234,* 235–236

Q

Quinoa
    adding to Tabbouleh, 224
    Red, and Potato Salad,
        Peruvian, 225–227, *226*
    for Salad, 108

R

Radicchio
    The Big Crunchy Autumn
        Vibes Salad, *158,* 159
    Crunchy Eggplant Parm Salad,
        206, 207–208
    Greek Golden Fava Salad
        Pita, *240,* 241–242
    Lazy Seitan Gyro Spinach
        Salad, 204–205, *206*
Radish(es)
    Avocado Salad, White Bean
        and Seitan Green Posole
        with, *272,* 273–274
    The Bright and Spicy Spring
        Asparagus Salad,
        151–152, *153*
    Korean Shiitake Bacon Salad
        Rice Bowl, 219–221, *220*
    Roasted Cabbage Steak with
        Peanut Sauce and Fried
        Shallots, 186–187
    Veggie Noodle Pho with Micro
        Bahn Mi Salad, 267–268
Ranch Dressings
    Sriracha Cilantro, 40, *41*
    Sunflower, *36,* 37–38, *49*
Rice
    Black, and Kabocha Salad,
        195–196, *197*
    The Bold and Bountiful Winter
        Salad, 160, *161*
    Bowl, Korean Shiitake Bacon
        Salad, 219–221, *220*
    Brown, Peanut Avocado
        Crunch Bowl, *210,* 211
    General Tso's Tofu and
        Broccoli Salad, *184,*
        185
    Peanut Avocado Brown Rice
        Crunch Bowl, *210,* 211
    Red Lentil Khichdi with Two
        Chutneys, 269–271
    Salad, 105
    Steamed Sticky, 215
    Sticky, Spicy Cucumber and

    Curry Tofu Salad with,
        212–215, *213*
Rice vinegar, 12
Root Bacon, 127–128, *129*

S

Salads
    assembling, 3–4
    fully dressed, refrigerating, 21
    green, crispy, crunchy, chewy,
        list of, x
    mise en place for, 4
    paired with soups, list of, xi
    pasta and grain, list of, xi
    preparing, with a scale, 19
    roasted, grilled, and hearty, list
        of, x–xi
Salad spinners, 9
Salt, 12, 13, 263
Salt, Pepper, and Vinegar
    Coconut Chips, 138
Salted Lemon Pepper Dressing, 47
Salted Lemons, 64–65
Sandwiches
    Chic Melts, *171,* 172
Sauces
    storing, 21
    Turmeric Tahini Miso, 44
Seaweeds
    about, 12
    The Chickpea of the Sea, 172
    Korean Shiitake Bacon Salad
        Rice Bowl, 219–221, *220*
    Peanut Avocado Brown Rice
        Crunch Bowl, *210,* 211
    Sun and Sea Sunflower
        Caesar Dressing, 39
Seed(s). *See also specific seeds*
    for creamy dairy-free
        dressings, 28
    and Nuts, Bacon Crunch,
        120–121
    for recipes, 11
    Seedy Garlic Bread Croutons,
        139–140

Seitan
about, 13, 74
The Bold and Bountiful Winter
Salad, 160, *161*
Cutlets, Steamed, 81–82
Gyro-Flavored, 204–205, *206*
Gyro Spinach Salad, Lazy,
204–205, *206*
Marinated Pan-Fried, 78
Protein-Packed Salad for
Breakfast, *190,* 191
Restaurant-Style Entrée
Caesar, 164
Roasted Cabbage Steak with
Peanut Sauce and Fried
Shallots, 186–187
and White Bean Green Posole
with Avocado Radish
Salad, *272,* 273–274
Sesame Dressing, Deep Dark, 55
Sesame seeds
Baby Carrot Ginger Soup with
Sesame Slaw, 260–261
black, about, 12
Korean Shiitake Bacon Salad
Rice Bowl, 219–221, *220*
Savory Sesame Tamari
Marinade, 85
Seedy Garlic Bread Croutons,
139–140
Sweet, Salty, Nutty Gomasio,
148
Sesame Slaw, Baby Carrot
Ginger Soup with,
260–261
Sesame Tamari Marinade, Savory,
85
7-Spice Peanuts, 111
Shallot(s)
Crispy Lime-and-Salt, 135
Fried, and Peanut Sauce,
Roasted Cabbage Steak
with, 186–187
Maple Mustard Vinaigrette, 70
Soups
Baby Carrot Ginger, with
Sesame Slaw, 260–261

Buffalo Tomato, with Kale
Caesar Salad, 250, *251*
Cauliflower, Creamy, with
Apple Walnut Salad,
254–256, *255*
Cranberry Bean and Pasta
Stew with Fennel Slaw,
262–263
Ethiopian Red Lentils with
Butternut and Avocado
Collard Salad, 257–259,
258
Green Again, with Tahini Miso
Slaw, 252, 253
Potato Leek, with Broccoli
Gremolata, 247–249, *248*
Red Lentil Khichdi with Two
Chutneys, 269–271
storing, 21
Thai Peanut Curry with Quick
Cucumber Pickles, *264,*
265–266
Veggie Noodle Pho with Micro
Bahn Mi Salad, 267–268
White Bean and Seitan Green
Posole with Avocado
Radish Salad, *272,*
273–274
Soy-free recipes, ingredient
swaps for, 21
Spices, 11
Spinach
All-Day Breakfast Nacho
Salad Bowl, 192–194,
193
Korean Shiitake Bacon Salad
Rice Bowl, 219–221, *220*
Pepita Greenest Goddess
Dressing, 51
Protein-Packed Salad for
Breakfast, *190,* 191
Seitan Gyro Salad, Lazy,
204–205, *206*
White Bean and Seitan Green
Posole with Avocado
Radish Salad, *272,*
273–274

Zhug Dressing, 198–200, *199*
Split peas
Greek Golden Fava Salad
Pita, *240,* 241–242
Red Lentil Khichdi with Two
Chutneys, 269–271
Squash. *See also* Zucchini
Butternut, Buffalo Tofu, and
Kale Bowl, 176, *177*
Ethiopian Red Lentils with
Butternut and Avocado
Collard Salad, 257–259,
258
Kabocha and Black Rice
Salad, 195–196, *197*
Protein-Packed Salad for
Breakfast, *190,* 191
Roasted Ratatouille Salad
with Romesco Dressing,
201–203, *202*
roasting directions, 191
Spaghetti, Thai Basil, with
Curry Tofu, 181–182, *183*
Sriracha
Cilantro Ranch Dressing, 40,
41
Orange Marinade, 90
Stew, Cranberry Bean and
Pasta, with Fennel Slaw,
262–263
Stir-Fried Salad, 218
Sumac powder, about, 12
Sunflower seeds
Nut-Free, Soy-Free Cheesy
Sunflower Crunch, 118,
119
soaking, 35
Sriracha Cilantro Ranch
Dressing, 40, *41*
Sun and Sea Sunflower
Caesar Dressing, 39
Sunflower Ranch Dressing,
36, 37–38, *49*
Toasted Sun and Pepita Parm,
110
Sweet Potato(es)
All-Day Breakfast Nacho

Salad Bowl, 192–194,
  193
White, Salad with Spinach
  Zhug Dressing, 198–200,
  199

T

Tabbouleh, Mustard Greens, with
  Almonds and Roasted
  Chickpeas, 222–224,
  223
Tahini
  Dressing, 43
  French Dressing, 45
  Mayo, 43
  Miso Marinade, 92
  Miso Slaw, Green Again Soup
    with, *252,* 253
  Turmeric Miso Sauce, 44
Tamari
  about, 13
  Sesame Marinade, Savory, 85
Tarragon Hemp Seed Dijon
  Dressing, 32
Tempeh
  about, 13, 74
  Blackened, Reuben Salad,
    178, 179
  The Bold and Bountiful Winter
    Salad, 160, *161*
  Kabocha and Black Rice
    Salad, 195–196, *197*
  Marinated or Baked, 77
  Orange Collard Greens, Corn,
    and Black-Eyed Peas,
    173–175, *174*
  Pastrami, Whole-Loaf
    Blackened, *96, 97*–98
  Peanut Avocado Brown Rice
    Crunch Bowl, *210,* 211
  Protein-Packed Salad for
    Breakfast, *190,* 191
  Restaurant-Style Entrée
    Caesar, 164
  Roasted Cabbage Steak with

Peanut Sauce and Fried
  Shallots, 186–187
Roasted Ratatouille Salad
  with Romesco Dressing,
  201–203, *202*
Thai Basil Spaghetti Squash with
  Curry Tofu, 181–182, *183*
Thai Peanut Curry with Quick
  Cucumber Pickles, *264,*
  265–266
Tofu
  about, 13, 74
  All-Day Breakfast Nacho
    Salad Bowl, 192–194,
    193
  The Big Crunchy Autumn
    Vibes Salad, *158,* 159
  Bites, Oven-Fried Breakfast,
    95
  The Bold and Bountiful Winter
    Salad, 160, *161*
  The Bright and Spicy Spring
    Asparagus Salad,
    151–152, *153*
  and Broccoli Salad, General
    Tso's, *184,* 185
  Buffalo, Butternut Squash, and
    Kale Bowl, 176, *177*
  cooked, storing, 21
  Curry, Thai Basil Spaghetti
    Squash with, 181–182,
    183
  Curry and Cucumber Salad,
    Spicy, with Sticky Rice,
    212–215, *213*
  freezing, 76
  Fried or Grilled, 76
  Kabocha and Black Rice
    Salad, 195–196, *197*
  Korean Shiitake Bacon Salad
    Rice Bowl, 219–221,
    220
  Marinated Baked, 75
  Mustard Greens Tabbouleh
    with Almonds and
    Roasted Chickpeas,
    222–224, *223*

Peanut Avocado Brown Rice
  Crunch Bowl, *210,* 211
Peking, Kelp Noodle Salad,
  218
Peking-Roasted, Noodle
  Salad, *216,* 217–218
Peruvian Potato and Red
  Quinoa Salad, 225–227,
  226
pressing, 76
Protein-Packed Salad for
  Breakfast, *190,* 191
ready-to-eat flavored, 80
Restaurant-Style Entrée
  Caesar, 164
Roasted Cabbage Steak with
  Peanut Sauce and Fried
  Shallots, 186–187
Roasted Ratatouille Salad
  with Romesco Dressing,
  201–203, *202*
Sriracha, Lettuce Wraps with
  Peanut Dressing, *168,*
  169
Sriracha Ranch Salad Party,
  165–166, *167*
Thai Peanut Curry with Quick
  Cucumber Pickles, *264,*
  265–266
Veggie Noodle Pho with Micro
  Bahn Mi Salad, 267–268
White Sweet Potato Salad
  with Spinach Zhug
  Dressing, 198–200, *199*
Za'atar, 92
Tomato(es)
  All-Day Breakfast Nacho
    Salad Bowl, 192–194,
    193
  Crunchy Eggplant Parm Salad,
    206, 207–208
  Greek Golden Fava Salad
    Pita, *240,* 241–242
  Lazy Seitan Gyro Spinach
    Salad, 204–205, *206*
  Mustard Greens Tabbouleh
    with Almonds and

Roasted Chickpeas, 222–224, *223*
New Catalina Dressing, 62, *63*
Pizza Panzanella with Beet Prosciutto, *234,* 235–236
Roasted, Chickpea Pasta Salad, 231–232, *233*
Roasted Pico de Gallo Dressing, 59
Roasted Ratatouille Salad with Romesco Dressing, 201–203, *202*
Soup, Buffalo, with Kale Caesar Salad, 250, *251*
Sriracha Ranch Salad Party, 165–166, *167*
Sun-Dried, Dressing, 60
Zucchini and Chickpea Fattoush Salad, 237–238, *239*
Tongs, 9
Topping recipes, list of, ix–x
Tortillas
 All-Day Breakfast Nacho Salad Bowl, 192–194, *193*
 Wheat, Toasted, 194
 White Bean and Seitan Green Posole with Avocado Radish Salad, *272, 273*–274
Turmeric
 Coconut Lime Chips, 138
 Tahini Miso Sauce, 44

V

Vegetable peelers, 8
Vegetables. *See also specific vegetables*
 roasted, storing, 21
 storing, 20
Veggie Noodle(s)
 buying, 268
 Pho with Micro Bahn Mi Salad, 267–268
 spiralizing, 268
Vinaigrettes
 Balsamic Dijon, 71
 Bright & Tangy Lemon Maple, 68
 Keep It Simple, 67
 Maple Mustard Shallot, 70
 Orange Balsamic, The Best, 72
 Oregano Garlic Lemon, 69
 Pomegranate, 69
Vinegars, 11, 12

W

Walnut(s)
 Apple Salad, Creamy Cauliflower Soup with, 254–256, *255*
 The Bright and Spicy Spring Asparagus Salad, 151–152, *153*
 Caesar, *122,* 123

Wasabi Miso Lime Dressing, 56
Watercress
 Kabocha and Black Rice Salad, 195–196, *197*
 Pepita Greenest Goddess Dressing, 51
White Balsamic Dressing, 69
Wraps
 Chickpea Pickle Collard, 170–172, *171*
 Sriracha Tofu Lettuce, with Peanut Dressing, *168,* 169

Y

Y-shaped peelers, 8
Yuba, Marinated Roasted, 79

Z

Za'atar Tofu, 92
Zhug Dressing, 198–200, *199*
Zucchini
 and Chickpea Fattoush Salad, 237–238, *239*
 Roasted Ratatouille Salad with Romesco Dressing, 201–203, *202*